Springer Series on Geriatric Nursing

Mathy D. Mezey, RN, EdD, FAAN, Series Editor
New York University Division of Nursing

1992 **Critical Care Nursing of the Elderly**
Terry T. Fulmer, RN, PhD, FAAN, and Mary K. Walker, PhD, RN, FAAN

1993 **Health Assessment of the Older Individual, Second Edition**
Mathy Doval Mezey, RN, EdD, FAAN, Shirlee Ann Stokes, RN, EdD, FAAN, and Louise Hartnett Rauckhorst, RNC, ANP, EdD

1994 **Nurse–Physician Collaboration: Care of Adults and the Elderly**
Eugenia L. Siegler, MD, and Fay W. Whitney, PhD, RN, FAAN

1995 **Strengthening Ge[...]**
Terry T. Fulm[...]), RN, Cs

1996 **Gerontology Re[...]**
Elizabeth Ch[...] r, DEd, RN, CRNP

1998 **Restraint-Fre[...] rs**
Neville E. S[...] binson, PhD, RN, J[...] Evans, DNSc, RN, [...]

1998 **Home Care fo[...] aregiv-ers—Text an[...]**
Mary Ann R[...]

Neville E. Strumpf, PhD, RN, C, FAAN, is an Associate Professor in the School of Nursing at the University of Pennsylvania and holds the Doris Schwartz Term Chair in Gerontological Nursing. She is Director of the Center for Gerontologic Nursing Science and of the Gerontological Nurse Practitioner Program. Dr. Strumpf has been widely recognized for work dedicated to restraint-free care in hospitals and nursing homes, including being honored with the prestigious Baxter Foundation Episteme Award in 1995. Dr. Strumpf has served as principal investigator on numerous government and foundation research and program grants, has written many articles and book chapters, and has lectured widely both nationally and internationally on care of older adults. She serves on many boards and advisory panels related to quality care for the aging, has been honored by the American Nurses' Association, New York University, and Sigma Theta Tau.

Joanne Patterson Robinson, PhD, RN, CS, is an Assistant Professor in the College of Nursing at Rutgers, The State University of New Jersey. Dr. Robinson served as a clinical director for the College's Robert Wood Johnson Foundation Teaching Nursing Home Project from 1983 to 1988. During doctoral study at the University of Pennsylvania School of Nursing, Dr. Robinson assisted Drs. Lois Evans and Neville Strumpf as the gerontologic nurse specialist in the NIA-funded clinical trial on restraint reduction in nursing homes. In 1995, she was honored by the Clinical Medicine Section of the Gerontological Society of America for her NINR-funded study of responses of institutionalized older adults to urinary incontinence. Dr. Robinson has authored or co-authored a variety of articles in the areas of restraint reduction, urinary incontinence, nursing practice in nursing homes, and professional nursing issues. She has spoken on gerontological nursing topics at numerous local and national conferences, and serves on two advisory boards for the New Jersey Department of Health and Senior Services.

Joan Stockman Wagner, MSN, CRNP, is a Senior Manager at The Whitman Group, America's SeniorCare Specialist located in Huntingdon Valley, PA. Ms. Wagner is a certified geriatric nurse practitioner with extensive nursing experience caring directly for older adults. She is recognized for her work in educating health professionals about the care of older adults both nationally and internationally. Ms. Wagner has presented educational programs to acute care and hospital-based nursing facility staff, educational institutions, and various gerontology groups and is involved in gerontologic product and resource development. Ms. Wagner has been a contributing author to several publications related to clinical practice issues.

Lois K. Evans, DNSc, RN, FAAN, holds the Viola MacInnes/Independence Chair in Nursing at the University of Pennsylvania School of Nursing where she is a professor and directs the School's Academic Nursing Practices. Dr. Evans directed a Robert Wood Johnson Foundation Teaching Nursing Home project, and has directed graduate programs in gerontologic and geropsychiatric nursing. In 1995, she received the prestigious Baxter Foundation Episteme Award for research on physical restraint in hospitals and nursing homes. Currently, Dr. Evans is providing leadership in the development and implementation of a model of academic nursing practice in a broad range of community-focused services.

Restraint-Free Care

Individualized Approaches for Frail Elders

Neville E. Strumpf, PhD, RN, C, FAAN
Joanne Patterson Robinson, PhD, RN
Joan Stockman Wagner, MSN, CRNP
Lois K. Evans, DNSc, RN, FAAN

Springer Publishing Company

Springer Publishing Company, Inc.
536 Broadway
New York, NY 10012-3955

Cover design by Janet Joachim
Acquisitions Editor: Ruth Chasek
Production Editor: Helen Song

01 02 / 4 3

Library of Congress Cataloging-in-Publication Data

Restraint-free care : individualized approaches for frail elders / by
Neville E. Strumpf . . . [et al.].
p. cm. -- (Springer series on geriatric nursing)
Includes bibliographical references and index.
ISBN 0-8261-1215-3
1. Nursing home care. 2. Nursing homes patients--Restraint. 3. Frail elderly--Nursing home care. I. Strumpf, Neville E. II. Series.
[DNLM: 1. Geriatric Nursing--methods. 2. Frail Elderly. 3. Restraint, Physical. 4. Patient Care Planning. 5. Nursing Homes. WY 152R436 1998]
RC954.3.R47 1998
362.1'6--dc21
DNLM/DLC
for Library of Congress 98-29833
CIP

Printed in the United States of America

For Doris Schwartz
and Carter Williams,
who provided wisdom, courage,
and inspiration for this work

Contents

Contributors

Roseanne Hanlon Rafter, MSN, RN, CS, CRRN, is a Gerontological Clinical Specialist with 13 years of experience in critical care. She has developed and implemented restraint reduction programs in multiple settings. She received the First Annual Springer award for her work in Restraint Reduction in 1993. Currently, she is a consultant with The Whitman Group, America's SeniorCare Specialist located in Huntingdon Valley, PA.

Pamela M. Zisselman, MSN, CRNP, is a geriatric nurse practitioner in the Department of Family Medicine, Thomas Jefferson University Hospital in Philadelphia. She is also a consultant on a geriatric psychiatry unit at the Wills Eye Hospital in Philadelphia and with the Gerontologic Nursing Consultation Service at the School of Nursing, University of Pennsylvania.

Preface

Restraint-Free Care: Individualized Approaches for Frail Elders is the culmination of a program of research begun by Lois Evans and Neville Strumpf in 1986, with inspiration from Doris Schwartz "to do something about the widespread problem of physical restraint." In 1990, with grant support from the Alzheimer's Association and from the National Institute on Aging for two studies aimed at reducing and eliminating physical restraints in nursing homes, we developed (with our collaborators, Joanne Patterson and Joan Wagner) a manual for teaching nursing home staff new ways to respond to resident behavior. Since then, the manual has undergone several evolutions in our thinking and in the presentation of content. The current manual represents a major revision of *Reducing Restraints: Individualized Approaches to Behavior*, prepared in 1992, and distributed widely by The Whitman Group, SeniorCare Specialists in Aging, in Huntingdon Valley, PA. This new edition has been written with both hospitalized elders and residents of nursing homes in mind.

In the debate over use of physical restraints, support has grown for their elimination based on lack of effectiveness and negative consequences with older adults. Although transition to restraint-free care is in progress, it is emerging as the standard for older adults in hospitals and nursing homes. Awareness has been heightened by recent Joint Commission on Accreditation of Healthcare Organizations (JCAHO) standards for restraint and seclusion, as well as FDA alerts and guidelines based on the OBRA '87 regulations for nursing homes. Nevertheless, standards and regulations alone do not bring about the necessary "paradigm shift" from viewing behavior as a problem to be controlled with physical restraints to viewing behavior as a communication of health state change or unmet need. Change in practice regarding interpretation and response to behavior comes about only as each organization or facility and their staff embrace a philosophy of restraint-free care, put in place policies and procedures that support changes in practice, and educate all care providers in the techniques of individualized care. This manual is designed to assist with that process and to disseminate research-based best practices for older adults.

A PHILOSOPHY OF INDIVIDUALIZED CARE

Most know the definition of a physical restraint: Any device (including siderails) placed on or near one's body to limit freedom of voluntary movement or normal access to one's own person. For us, however, physical restraints (and the inappropriate use of psychoactive drugs) are even more than that. They also symbolize a poor quality of care because of failure to address real needs of the person.

Our manual is framed by a philosophy of individualized care, which we believe to be the key to understanding older adults and to providing restraint-free care. The goals of individualized care include promoting comfort and safe mobility, optimizing function and independence, and achieving the greatest possible dignity and quality of life. Such care requires clinicians to make sense of behavior rather than to control responses of clients.

In this manual the reader will observe that "alternatives to restraints" are not discussed. In our view, the problem of restraint use can be resolved through careful assessment of the client, a focus on "making sense of behavior," and implementation of individualized interventions tailored to specific needs.

ORGANIZATION OF THE MANUAL

The manual is designed for anyone seeking information on individualized restraint-free care. It is organized in outline format to highlight critical material and to be readily adaptable as a quick reference for clinicians, or as an adjunct for teaching staff or educating administrators, board members, and consumers.

The manual is divided into seven chapters, each with a stated purpose, and a detailed content outline, bibliography, and appendixes. The first three chapters provide background on restraint use and lay the foundation for making changes in practice.

Chapter 1, "Achieving Restraint-Free Care," summarizes a decade of literature and research on feelings, beliefs and reasons associated with restraint use, myths and facts, and ethical considerations. In chapter 2, change processes are described, including groups to target, steps to follow, and clinical models in nursing homes and hospitals. The methods for "Making Sense of Behavior," the cornerstone of our approach to restraint-free care, are detailed in chapter 3. A three-part strategy for the clinical evaluation of behavior is given: Getting to know the person, analyzing the context or circumstances of the behavior, and determining meaning of the behavior.

Most often physical restraints are applied because of behavioral phenomena, falls, and interference with treatment. Chapters 4, 5, and 6 provide the tools for assessing these situations and arriving at solutions that are congruent with individualized restraint-free care.

In the final chapter, "Maintaining a Process of Change," we reiterate the importance of a systematic individualized assessment, describe ways to maintain momentum, and offer suggestions for modifying policy and procedures related to restraint use. We also include several case studies using the Behavior Log, a matrix of selected interventions, and a listing of other resources.

We remain deeply committed to the goal of restraint-free care for every older adult in any care setting. While we have clearly witnessed improvements toward achieving this goal, restraint-free care is, as yet, not a reality. In preparing this manual, and through disseminating this knowledge, we hope that our readers and ourselves will never know physical restraint in the 21st century.

Neville E. Strumpf
Lois K. Evans
Philadelphia, 1998

1

Achieving Restraint-Free Care

Neville E. Strumpf and Lois K. Evans

The Purpose of this Chapter is to:

1. Establish restraint-free care as the standard of care for older adults in all settings.
2. Identify common reasons cited for restraint use with older adults.
3. Describe untoward effects of physical restraints on older adults.
4. Provide background on ethical, legal, regulatory, and other standards related to use of restraints with older adults.
5. Summarize the philosophy of individualized restraint-free care and its application to older adults.

I. Impact of Physical Restraint on Older Adults and Their Nurses

A. Many feelings and responses to physical restraint have been expressed by older adults (Strumpf & Evans, 1988), including:

1. Anger: "I have done nothing to deserve this [restraints]. To think you fought a war—now I am a POW!"
2. Fear: "If there was a fire, I'd be caught. When someone is tied and chained in a fire, how will you save the person? How would I get out?"

3. Resistance: "The first time I was aware of the restraint was when I woke up. I tried to untie my hands to resist. I think any human being would."
4. Humiliation: "I couldn't move at all to do what I wanted or needed. I couldn't even bring my hands together. I felt like I was nailed to a cross."
5. Demoralization: "I felt like a dog and cried all night. It hurt me to be tied up. I felt like I was nobody, that I was dirt. It makes me cry to talk about it (tears). The hospital is worse than a jail."
6. Discomfort: "I felt it [the restraint] across my chest and I felt pain. I asked [the staff] to cut it off."
7. Resignation: "After a while I gave up; I became a mouse."
8. Denial: "I never had nothing like that [restraints]. That's for crazy people. I was never like that. You must be mistaken; maybe the nurses had me mixed up with someone else."
9. Agreement: "If I hadn't been tied down, I might have fallen. Here they only do it [apply restraints] for your protection. If a person objects, then he's lacking up there (points to head). The thing to do is forget it; any sane person shouldn't object."
10. Disagreement/Betrayal: "They told me I was confused when I was perfectly sane; when people are confused they do not need restraint; that drives them over the wall."

B. The following case example was provided by an older woman who was physically restrained during hospitalization. Many emotions are evident in her comments, which clearly demonstrate the need to explore restraint-free approaches to care.

> "I was taken by ambulance to the hospital emergency room because of palpitations; there I received lidocaine to which I was 'allergic.' Apparently it caused me to misbehave badly, and I tried to climb out of bed. I don't remember misbehaving, but I may have been deranged from all the pills they gave me. Normally I am spirited, but I am also good and obedient. Nevertheless, the nurse tied me down, like Jesus on the cross, by bandaging both wrists and ankles. As I lay there I wondered if His arms and legs had ached like mine. I said, 'My hands and ankles will swell.' It felt awful, I hurt, and I worried, 'What if I get leg cramps, what will I do then if I can't move?' It was miserable, not being able to move, and an awful shock. It was unfair of the hospital to tie me. I felt terrible, aching pain and numbness; I wonder now how I ate; no one fed me that I know of. And I don't think I slept at night. Because I am a cooperative person, I felt so resentful. Callers, including men friends, saw me like that and I lost something; I lost a little personal prestige. I was embarrassed, like a child placed

in a corner for being bad. I had been important, and well, and to be tied down in bed took a big toll." (Strumpf, Evans, & Schwartz, 1991).

C. Nurses and other direct caregivers also feel the impact of restraining another and voice many concerns (Strumpf & Evans, 1988). These include a range of feelings, among them:

1. Anxiety.
2. Sense of inadequacy.
3. Hopelessness or helplessness.
4. Frustration.
5. Anger with the client, other staff members, or conditions in the environment.
6. Fear, especially of personal injury by someone who is aggressive.
7. Guilt.
8. Satisfaction, e.g., the problem has been "handled."
9. Sense of being overwhelmed.
10. Repugnance, e.g., "I hate to restrain."

D. Listed below are comments from nurses responsible for the care of hospitalized older persons who were physically restrained. These statements reflect the ethical conflicts staff experience as they attempt to "protect clients from harm."

1. "I'd rather use a restraint than have her fall."
2. "I tell myself it's for their own safety. I can't allow myself to feel sorry for the patient."
3. "Sometimes it bothers me when the patient can't understand the need for restraint. I wonder if it's for his own good."
4. "It drives me crazy to restrain so many patients; I feel like a jailer rather than a nurse."
5. "Everyone hated to restrain him; he was such a nice man. But he seemed to accept it and he became used to it, which helped the staff."

II. Myths and Facts About Restraint Use

In a widely cited article, Evans and Strumpf (1990) exposed the myths and facts about restraint use. These are described below and summarized in Appendix A.

A. *Myth I*: "The old should be restrained because they are more likely to fall and seriously injure themselves." In fact, research suggests that:

1. Injuries can occur when restraints are used:

a. Many clients untie or attempt to remove restraints; numerous falls and injuries have occurred, especially from wheelchairs.
b. Bedrails, designed to enhance client safety, may in fact undermine it. Older clients often climb over rails with the intention of reaching the bathroom, and then fall to the floor from a greater height.
c. Use of restraints and bedrails can result in death. In recent years, restraining vests have caused strangulation or asphyxiation in hundreds of people.

2. In the United States, approaches to care of older adults have been dominated by undue emphasis on safety, particularly in instances of perceived risk for falls.

a. In the United Kingdom, falls are a more accepted occurrence in geriatric care settings:

(1) Promotion and maintenance of functional ability is the focus of care, i.e., restorative focus.
(2) Restrictions in activity are thought to present greater hazards than the risk of falls.
(3) Risk-taking is considered essential to successful rehabilitation and maintenance of independence and dignity.
(4) Falls are common, but serious injury rates are low and comparable to rates in the U.S.

b. A "safety first" approach, dominant in the U.S., may lead to loss of mobility and more restricted lives than necessary for older persons.

B. *Myth II*: "The moral duty to protect patients from harm requires restraint." In fact, research suggests that:

1. A physical restraint, which is meant to protect, has no known therapeutic value and in certain cases may actually be hazardous.
2. Untoward physical effects of restraint use with older adults include:

a. Skin trauma (e.g., tears, cuts, bruises).
b. Pressure ulcers.
c. Pneumonia and respiratory complications.
d. Incontinence.
e. Constipation.
f. Abnormal physiologic changes in electrolytes, metabolism, and blood volume (reduced circulatory volume).
g. Orthostatic hypotension.
h. Lower extremity edema.

i. Decreased muscle mass, tone, strength and endurance leading to loss of functional capacity.
j. Bone demineralization (e.g., fragility and increased risk of fracture).
k. Altered nutrition (e.g., restraint may contribute to inability or lack of desire to eat).
l. Nosocomial infection (e.g., pneumonia, urinary tract infections from immobility).
m. Cardiac stress (e.g., changes in blood pressure, pulse, exercise tolerance).
n. Serious physical injury.
o. Possible destruction of selected brain cells.
p. Death (from strangulation or asphyxiation).

3. Untoward psychosocial effects of restraint use with older adults include:

   a. Combativeness or aggressiveness.
   b. Anger.
   c. Fear of abandonment.
   d. Increased confusion.
   e. Social isolation.
   f. Dependency.
   g. Regression.
   h. Withdrawal.
   i. Loss of self-esteem.

C. *Myth III*: "Failure to restrain puts individuals and facilities at risk for legal liability." In fact:

   1. Federal (OBRA '87) and/or state regulations for nursing homes require that *restraints be imposed ONLY*:

      a. To ensure the physical safety of the resident or other residents.
      b. Upon the written order of a physician specifying duration and circumstances under which the restraints are to be used (except in emergency circumstances until such an order can be reasonably obtained).
      c. After assessment of the resident's capabilities, evaluation of less restrictive approaches, and ruling out in this instance the use of other interventions.
      d. After development of a schedule or plan of rehabilitative training to enable progressive removal of restraints or progressive use of less restrictive means, as indicated.

2. Revised Standards for Restraint and Seclusion developed by the Joint Commission on Accreditation of Healthcare Organizations (JCAHO) require that hospitals and other health care organizations create a physical, social, and cultural environment that:

    a. "Limits use of restraint and seclusion to clinically appropriate and adequately justified situations."
    b. "Reduces use of restraint and seclusion through preventive or alternative strategies."

3. Successful lawsuits based solely on failure to restrain appear to be rare or non-existent. Lawsuits involving use of restraints are increasing.
4. Care is judged against standards of practice (see Appendix B), specifying that:

    a. Behavior should trigger assessment and intervention aimed at individualized approaches to care without restraint.
    b. In the rare circumstance where a restraint is applied, this should only occur as a result of collaborative decision making among nurse, physician and other health team members. Such a decision should be the result of comprehensive assessment, case review, and sufficient evidence of attempted interventions. This decision must also incorporate informed participation and consent by patients/residents and families.
    c. Restraints are never used as a substitute for observation.
    d. If for any reason restraints are to be used, then use is as a short-term measure only and as a last resort. Any application of a physical restraint is to be done by properly trained staff who are keenly aware of the potential hazards. When short-term use is unavoidable, attention to comfort, safety, and needs for food, hydration, elimination, exercise, and social interaction are required. The client should be debriefed following the experience of restraint to prevent negative emotional consequences.

5. The gold standard of practice is restraint-free care. Evidence of restraint use reflects system failures and resistance to accepted standards of care.

    a. Restraint-free care is endorsed by the Task Force on Risk-Taking, Choice, and Control of the Gerontological Society of America (1994), as well as by the American Geriatrics Society (1995).
    b. Both groups support restraint-free care as the goal for care of older persons *in all settings*.

6. Components of successful restraint-free care are:

    a. Administrative commitment.
    b. Individualized approaches to care.
    c. Access to ongoing education and consultation.
    d. Comprehensive plan of care.
    e. Regular team meetings to discuss care.
    f. Knowledgeable staff and families.
    g. Consistent assignment of nursing staff.
    h. Stability among leadership staff.
    i. Relationships and rapport between care providers and care recipients.
    j. Home-like environment.

7. The best legal protection lies in providing people with individualized care and humane, respectful treatment consistent with current professional and regulatory standards.

D. *Myth IV*: "It doesn't really bother older people to be restrained." Field notes from research by Strumpf and Evans suggest that:

    1. Clients generally have negative feelings about restraint (See also I.A.).
    2. Clients often report profound awareness of the application of restraint:

        a. "I may not have remembered what the nurse told me [not to get out of bed], but I was fully aware of being tied. I didn't feel confused, but the nurse kept asking me if I was confused, and the longer I took to answer, I guess the more confused she thought I was."
        b. "It's hard to be in bed [restrained]; you can't move. It's terrible; you don't know what's going to happen. You look around and you hardly know where you are. It makes your mind go a little bit."

    3. People struggle to understand the reasons for application of a restraint.

E. *Myth V*: "We have to restrain because of inadequate staffing." In fact:

    1. Elimination or reduction of restraint use in many hospitals and nursing homes has been achieved without increases in staff.
    2. Improvement in functional status may be a positive outcome of eliminating or reducing restraint use:

        a. Improved functional status often means greater ability for self-care and less need for assistance.

b. Improved functional status enhances safe mobility.

3. Use of physical restraints increases the time to provide care (Phillips, Hawes, & Fries, 1993), since restraint use requires frequent:

   a. Inspection.
   b. Release.
   c. Exercise.
   d. Opportunity to use toilet, commode, bedpan, or urinal.
   e. Monitoring.
   f. Evaluation.

F. *Myth VI*: "No interventions for meeting client needs are available." In fact, research suggests that a range of individualized interventions in the following categories have eliminated physical restraints:

   1. Physiologic.
   2. Psychosocial.
   3. Activity.
   4. Environmental modification.

   Note: These interventions are discussed in greater detail in later chapters and examples are summarized in chapter 7, Appendix A.

III. Common Reasons for Restraint Use

Despite a growing body of empiric evidence reporting the harms of physical restraint, and even with legislative and regulatory mandates supporting minimal or no restraint, the practice continues.

A. Background

   1. Definition: A physical restraint is any device placed on or near the body which limits freedom of voluntary movement and free access to one's body. Examples include:

      a. Bedrails.
      b. Geriatric or recliner chairs with fixed tray tables.
      c. Vests.
      d. Wrist and ankle ties.
      e. Waist belts.
      f. Seat belts.
      g. Hand mitts.

   2. Prevalence of physical restraint use varies with:

a. Age (higher rates in the very old).
b. Functional status (higher rates in the very frail).
c. Cognitive level (higher rates with greater impairment).

3. Prior to implementation of OBRA '87 regulations, restraint use prevailed at rates of:

   a. 40% in skilled care facilities.
   b. 31% in intermediate care facilities.
   c. 34% among older adults in rehabilitation settings.
   d. 22% among older adults in acute care hospitals.

4. Subsequent to implementation of OBRA '87 regulations:

   a. Less than 20% of residents in nursing home facilities are restrained based on self-reports (HCFA, 1995).
   b. Percentages in acute care are unknown, but appear similar to 1990 levels.

B. Common Reasons for Restraint Use With Older Adults

   1. Protection from self-injury (e.g., falls, mobility in unsafe areas).
   2. Protection of others (e.g., from intrusion, aggression, or assault).
   3. Provision of necessary medical treatments (e.g., tube feedings, intravenous lines, urinary catheters).
   4. Perceived legal and family pressure.

C. Less common reasons include:

   1. Insufficient staff.
   2. Efficiency in "managing" behavior.

D. Frequent and common use of restraints permits the practice to become a norm, making reduction or elimination more difficult to achieve.

IV. Ethical Considerations Related to Restraint Use (see Appendix C)

In early discussions of restraint use, the emphasis, ethically, was on matters pertaining to restrictions of autonomy or to questions of beneficence. As empiric evidence has mounted for the harmful consequences of restraint, and the standard of care has shifted toward minimal or no restraint use, ethical arguments must now also consider the obligations of providers to assure that appropriate standards of care are delivered and maintained. In examining the various facets of restraint use, ethical discussions continue to focus on burdens, rights, and responsibilities, as summarized briefly below.

A. Burdens of restraint use for clients are many, including:

1. Physical consequences (as noted earlier).
2. Psychosocial consequences (as noted earlier).
3. Loss of freedom, control, and choice.

B. Protection of human rights in the context of restraint use requires that the rights of several parties be considered:

1. The client for whom the restraint is proposed.
2. Other clients in the facility.
3. Staff.
4. Family.

C. Specific rights of clients related to principles of autonomy, beneficence, and veracity must be considered. These include:

1. Freedom of choice, self-direction, independence.
2. Freedom from harm.
3. Freedom to take risks.
4. Right to be informed.
5. Right to be treated with respect.
6. Right to be treated as an individual.

V. Caregiver Responsibilities

A. Attend to the older adult's needs and preferences concerning care through:

1. Conversations with the client, family, friends, and care providers to elicit information about usual routines for activities of daily living.
2. Exploration of advance directives, and systematic communication of the client's wishes to all members of the health care team.
3. Obtaining a social and/or values history to determine the appropriate context for providing care.
4. Providing individualized care (refer to chapter 3).

B. Educate older adults and family members about the risks and burdens of restraint use.
C. Make collaborative decisions concerning provision of care with the older adult and family.
D. Document decision-making processes in the health care record.

E. At the core of all ethical care is compassionate treatment focused on the maintenance of human dignity.

VI. Summary

The philosophy of restraint-free care assumes that each person be cared for as a separate and unique individual; that people's rights be respected; that care be directed toward the maintenance of dignity, autonomy, self-esteem, and physical well-being; and that all persons be assured the highest possible quality of life. Restraint use is inconsistent with a philosophy of individualized care. As health care institutions move toward restraint-free care, key points to remember are that:

A. Restraint-free care is emerging as the gold standard of practice in care of older adults.
B. Legal precedent suggests that provision of individualized care based on standards of practice and humane, respectful, relationship-based treatment is key to preventing claims of malpractice.
C. Physical restraints are often used because people believe that they are effective and that other interventions are not possible.
D. Restraints do not remove the risk of falls and injuries and may, in fact, intensify the seriousness of injuries and other hazards, including death.
E. Being restrained is uncomfortable and has serious consequences for older adults and staff.
F. Use of physical restraint is inconsistent with a philosophy of individualized care. The practice should play no part in the care of older persons in institutional or community settings.

Bibliography

American Geriatrics Society. (1995). *American Geriatrics Society (AGS) clinical practice statement: The use of restraints*. New York, NY: Author.

Braun, J. A. (1998). Legal aspects of physical restraint use in nursing homes. *The Health Lawyer, 10*(3), 20, 10–16.

Bryant, H., & Fernald, L. (1997). Nursing knowledge and use of restraint alternatives: Acute and chronic care. *Geriatric Nursing, 18*, 57–60.

Burlington, D. B. (1995). *FDA Safety Alert: Entrapment hazards with hospital bed side rails*. Washington, DC: Food and Drug Administration, Public Health Service, Department of Health & Human Services.

Burton, L. C., German, P. S., Rovner, B. W., & Brant, L. J. (1992). Physical restraint use and cognitive decline among nursing home residents. *Journal of the American Geriatrics Society, 40*, 811–816.

Capezuti, E. (1991). Restraint research. *Oasis, 8*(3), 5.
Capezuti, E., Evans, L. K., Strumpf, N. E., & Maislin, G. (1996). Physical restraint use and falls in nursing home residents. *Journal of the American Geriatrics Society, 44,* 627–633.
Capezuti, E., Strumpf, N. E., Evans, L. K., Grisso, J. A., & Maislin, G. (1998). The relationship between physical restraint removal and falls and injuries among nursing home residents. *Journal of Gerontology: Medical Sciences, 53A,* M47–M52.
Castle, N. G., Fogel, B., & Mor, V. (1997). Risk factors for physical restraint use in nursing homes: Pre- and post-implementation of the Nursing Home Reform Act. *The Gerontologist, 37,* 737–747.
Castle, N. G., & Mor, V. (1998). Physical restraints in nursing homes: A review of the literature since the nursing home reform act of 1987. *Medical Care Research and Review, 55*(2), 139–170.
Conely, L., & Campbell, L. (1991). The use of restraints in caring for the elderly: Realities, consequences, and alternatives. *Nurse Practitioner, 16*, 48–52.
Creditor, M. C. (1993). Hazards of hospitalization of the elderly. *Annals of Internal Medicine, 118*, 219–223.
Difabio, S. (1981). Nurses' reactions to restraining patients. *American Journal of Nursing, 81*, 973–975.
DiMaio, J. M., Dana, S. E., & Bux, R. C. (1986). Deaths caused by restraint vests [Letter to the editor]. *The New England Journal of Medicine, 255*, 905.
Dube, A. H., & Mitchell, E. K. (1986). Accidental strangulation from vest restraints. *Journal of the American Medical Association, 256*, 2725–2726.
Dunbar, J. (1993, November). *Restraint review.* (Available from Joan Dunbar, The Jewish Home and Hospital for the Aged, 120 West 106th Street, New York, NY 10025).
Ejaz, F. K., Jones, J. A., & Rose, M. S. (1994). Falls among nursing home residents: An examination of incident reports before and after restraint reduction programs. *Journal of the American Geriatrics Society, 42*, 960–964.
Evans, L. K. (1996). Knowing the patient: The route to individualized care. *Journal of Gerontological Nursing, 22*(3), 15–19.
Evans, L., & Strumpf, N. (1987). Patterns of restraint: A cross-cultural view. *The Gerontologist, 27*, (Special Issue), 272A–273A.
Evans, L., & Strumpf, N. (1990). Myths about elder restraint. *Image: Journal of Nursing Scholarship, 22*, 124–128.
Evans, L., Strumpf, N., & Williams, C. (1991). Redefining a standard of care for frail older people: Alternatives to routine physical restraint. In P. Katz, R. Kane, & M. Mezey (Eds.), *Advances in long term care, I.* New York: Springer Publishing Co., 81–108.
Evans, L., Strumpf, N., & Williams, C. (1992). Limiting restraints: A prerequisite for independent functioning. In E. Calkins, A. Ford, & P. Katz (Eds.), *Practice of geriatrics*, 2nd ed. Philadelphia: Saunders.
Fletcher, K. (1996). Use of restraints in the elderly. *AACN Clinical Issues, 7*, 611–620.
Frengley, J. D., & Mion, L. C. (1986). Incidence of physical restraints on acute general medical wards. *Journal of the American Geriatrics Society, 34*, 565–568.
Gerontological Society of America. (1994). *Task force on risk-taking, choice and control: The case of physical restraint.* Washington, DC: Author.
Happ, M. B., Williams, C. C., Strumpf, N. E., & Burger, S. G. (1996). Individualized care for frail elders: Theory and practice. *Journal of Gerontological Nursing, 22*(3), 6–14.
Hardin, S. B., Magee, R., Vinson, M. H., Owen, M., Hyatt, E., & Stratmann, D. (1993). Patient and family perception of restraints. *Journal of Holistic Nursing, 11*, 383–397.

Health Care Financing Administration. (1990, October 1). Survey procedures and interpretive guidelines for skilled and intermediate care facilities (Appendix P). In *State operations manual: Provider certification*. Washington, DC: U.S. Government Printing Office.

Health Care Financing Administration. (1988). *Medicare/Medicaid Nursing Home Information: 1987–1988*. Washington, DC: U.S. Government Printing Office.

Janelli, L. M., Scherer, Y. K., Kanski, G. W., & Neary, M. A. (1991). What nursing staff members really know about physical restraints. *Rehabilitation Nursing, 16*, 345–348.

Joint Commission on Accreditation of Healthcare Organizations. (1996). Revised standards and scoring guidelines for restraint and seclusion (Appendix D). In *Comprehensive accreditation manual for hospitals*. Oakbrook Terrace, IL: Author.

Kapp, M. B. (1992). Nursing home restraints and legal liability: Merging the standard of care and industry practice. *Journal of Legal Medicine, 13*, 1–32.

Kapp, M. B. (1994). Physical restraints in hospitals: Risk management's reduction role. *Journal of Healthcare Risk Management, 14*, 3–8.

Kapp, M. B. (1996). Physical restraint use in critical care: Legal issues. *AACN Clinical Issues, 7*, 579–584.

Lofgren, R. P., MacPherson, D. S., Granieri, R., Myllenbeck, S., & Sprafka, J. M. (1989). Mechanical restraints on the medical wards: Are protective devices safe? *American Journal of Public Health, 79*, 735–738.

Mahoney, D. F. (1995). Analysis of restraint free nursing homes. *Image: Journal of Nursing Scholarship, 27*, 155–160.

McLardy-Smith, P., Burge, P., & Watson, N. (1986). Ischaemic contracture of the intrinsic muscles of the hands: A hazard of restraint. *Journal of Hand Surgery, 11-B*(1), 65–67.

Miles, S., & Irvine, P. (1992). Deaths caused by physical restraints. *The Gerontologist, 32*, 762–766.

Mion, L., Frengley, J. D., & Adams, M. (1986). Nursing patients 75 years and older. *Nursing Management, 17*(9), 24–28.

Mion, L. C., & Strumpf, N. E. (1994). Use of physical restraints in the hospital setting: Implications for the nurse. *Geriatric Nursing, 15*(3), 127–132.

Mitchell-Pederson, L., Edmund, L., Fingerote, E., & Powell, C. (1985). Let's untie the elderly. *Ontario Association of Homes for the Aged Quarterly, 21*(10), 10–14.

Morse, J. M., & McHutchion, E. (1991). Releasing restraints: Providing safe care for the elderly. *Research in Nursing & Health, 14*, 187–196.

Moss, R. J., & Lapuma, J. (1991). The ethics of mechanical restraints. *Hastings Center Report*, January/February, 22–25.

Ney, A. (1993, April 27). Death in personal care home ruled an accident. *Citizen Voice*, pp. 4, 24.

Omnibus Budget Reconciliation Act [OBRA] of 1987. P.L. 100-203. Subtitle C. The Nursing Home Reform Act. 42 U.S.C. 1395i-3(a)-(h) (Medicare); 13966v(a)-(h) Medicaid.

Papougenis, D. (1989). What's the law? *Untie the Elderly, 1*(1), 3.

Parker, K., & Miles, S. N. (1997). Deaths caused by bedrails. *Journal of the American Geriatrics Society, 45*, 797–802.

Powell, C., Mitchell-Pederson, L., Fingerote, E., & Edmund, L. (1989). Freedom from restraint: Consequences of reducing physical restraints in the management of the elderly. *Canadian Medical Association Journal, 141*, 561–563.

Phillips, C. D., Hawes, C., & Fries, B. E. (1993). Reducing the use of physical restraints in nursing homes: Will it increase costs? *American Journal of Public Health, 83*, 342–348.

Quinn, C. A. (1993). Nurses' perception about physical restraints. *Western Journal of Nursing Research, 15*, 148–162.

Rader, J., Semradek, J., McKenzie, D., & McMahon, M. (1992). Restraint strategies: Reducing restraints in Oregon's long-term care facilities. *Journal of Gerontological Nursing, 18*(11), 49–56.

Reigle, J. (1996). The ethics of physical restraints in critical care. *AACN Clinical Issues, 7*, 585–591.

Robbins, L., Boyko, E., Lane, J., Cooper, D., & Jahnigen, D. (1987). Binding the elderly: A prospective study of the use of mechanical restraints in an acute care hospital. *Journal of the American Geriatrics Society, 35*, 2909–296.

Robinson, B. E., Sucholeiki, R., & Schocken, D. D. (1993). Sudden death and resisted mechanical restraint: A case report. *Journal of the American Geriatrics Society, 41*, 424–425.

Rowles, G. D., & High, D. M. (1996). Individualizing care: Family roles in nursing home decision-making. *Journal of Gerontological Nursing, 22*(3), 20–25.

Scott, T. F., & Gross, J. A. (1989). Brachial plexus injury due to vest restraints [Letter to the editor]. *New England Journal of Medicine, 320*, 598.

Sexton, T. R., Leiken, A. M., Sleeper, S., & Coburn, A. F. (1989). The impact of prospective reimbursement on nursing home efficiency. *Medical Care, 27*(2), 154–163.

Skeen, M. B., Rozear, M. P., & Morgenlander, J. C. (1992, November 1). Posey palsy [Letter to the editor]. *Annals of Internal Medicine, 117*(9), 795.

Stilwell, E. (1991). Nurses' education related to the use of restraints. *Journal of Gerontological Nursing, 17*(2), 23–26.

Strumpf, N. E., & Evans, L. K. (1988). Physical restraint of the hospitalized elderly: Perceptions of patients and nurses. *Nursing Research, 37*(3), 132–137.

Strumpf, N. E., & Evans, L. K. (1991). The ethical problems of prolonged physical restraint. *Journal of Gerontological Nursing, 17*(2), 27–30.

Strumpf, N. E., Evans, L. K., & Schwartz, D. (1991). Physical restraint of older people. In C. Chenitz, S. Stone, & S. Salisbury (Eds.), pp. 329–344. *The clinical practice of gerontological nursing*. Philadelphia: Saunders.

Strumpf, N. E., Evans, L. K., & Schwartz, D. (1990). Restraint free care: From dream to reality. *Geriatric Nursing, 11*(3), 122–124.

Strumpf, N. E., & Tomes, N. (1993). Restraining the troublesome patient: A historical perspective on a contemporary debate. *Nursing History Review, 1*, 3–24.

Sullivan-Marx, E. M. (1995). Psychological responses to physical restraint use in older adults. *Journal of Psychosocial Nursing, 33*(6), 20–25.

Sullivan-Marx, E. M., & Strumpf, N. E. (1996). Restraint free care for acutely ill patients in the hospital. *AACN Clinical Issues, 7*, 572–578.

Sullivan-Marx, E. M., Strumpf, N. E., & Evans, L. K. (in press). Restraint free care of the elderly. In S. Salisbury, J. T. Stone, & J. Wyman (Eds.), *Clinical gerontological nursing: A guide for advanced practice*. Philadelphia: W. B. Saunders.

Tinetti, M. E., Liu, W. L., Marottoli, R. A., & Ginter, S. F. (1991). Mechanical restraint use among residents of skilled nursing facilities: Prevalence, patterns, and predictors. *Journal of the American Medical Association, 265*, 468–471.

Tinetti, M. E., Liu, W. L., & Ginter, S. F. (1992). Mechanical restraint use and fall-related injuries among residents of skilled nursing facilities. *Annals of Internal Medicine, 116*, 369–374.

Walshe, A., & Rosen, H. (1979). A study of patient falls from bed. *Journal of Nursing Administration, 9*(5), 31–35.

Weick, M. D. (1992). Physical restraints: An FDA update. *American Journal of Nursing, 92*(11), 74–80.

Yarmesch, M., & Sheafor, M. (1984). The decision to restrain. *Geriatric Nursing, 11*, 242–244.

Appendix A

Myths and Facts About Physical Restraint Use

	MYTH	FACT
I.	**"The old should be restrained because they are more likely to fall and seriously injure themselves."**	• Restraints do not remove the risk of falls and serious injuries.
II.	**"The moral duty to protect from harm requires restraint."**	• Physical restraints, applied in the belief that they protect clients, have no known therapeutic value, and may be hazardous. • "Protecting" older adults with physical restraints places them at risk for numerous short- and long-term physical, psychological, and behavioral consequences.
III.	**"Failure to restrain puts individuals and facilities at risk for legal liability."**	• Federal and state regulations restrict use of physical and chemical restraints for nursing home residents; JCAHO guidelines limit use of restraint and seclusion in hospitals and other health care organizations. • To hold a professional liable requires evidence that minimum standards of practice have been ignored or violated.

IV.	**"It doesn't really bother older people to be restrained."**	• Interviews with restrained older people reveal feelings ranging from anger, fear, humiliation, resistance, discomfort, demoralization, resignation, and denial.
V.	**"We have to restrain because of inadequate staffing."**	• Many facilities have eliminated or reduced restraint use, without increases in staffing. • More time is required to care for restrained clients, who must receive frequent inspection, release, exercise, use of toilet, monitoring, and evaluation than those who are not restrained.
VI.	**"No interventions, other than physical restraint, are available."**	• Interventions for meeting client needs *are* available and have been successful in eliminating physical restraints. • Four categories of individualized interventions include: — Physiologic approaches — Psychosocial approaches — Activity and exercise programs — Environmental modification

Adapted from: Evans, L., & Strumpf, N. (1990). Myths about elder restraint. *Image: Journal of Nursing Scholarship, 22*, 124–128.

Appendix B

Standards of Practice Related to Physical Restraint Use

1. Behavior should trigger assessment and intervention aimed at individualized approaches to care without restraint.
2. In the rare circumstance where a restraint is applied, this should only occur as a result of collaborative decision making among nurse, physician and other health team members. Such a decision should be the result of comprehensive assessment, case review, and sufficient evidence of attempted interventions. This decision must also incorporate informed participation and consent by patients/residents and families.
3. Restraints are never used as a substitute for observation.
4. If for any reason restraints are to be used, then use is as a short-term measure and only as a *last resort*. Any application of a physical restraint is to be done by properly trained staff who are keenly aware of the potential hazards. When short-term use is unavoidable, attention to comfort, safety, and needs for food, hydration, elimination, exercise, and social interaction are required. The client should be debriefed following the experience of restraint to prevent negative emotional consequences.

Appendix C

Ethical Considerations Related to Physical Restraint Use

BURDENS OF RESTRAINT USE FOR CLIENTS:

- Physical consequences.
- Psychosocial consequences.
- Loss of freedom, control and choice.

PARTIES WHO MUST BE CONSIDERED:

- The client for whom the restraint is proposed.
- Other clients in the facility.
- Staff.
- Family.

SPECIFIC RIGHTS OF CLIENTS:

- Freedom of choice and self-direction.
- Freedom from harm.
- Freedom to take risks.
- Right to be informed.
- Right to be treated with respect.
- Right to be treated as an individual.

2

Implementing a Process of Change

Joanne Patterson Robinson and Neville E. Strumpf

The Purpose of this Chapter is to:

Outline a process of change as it relates to restraint-free care.

I. Process of Change

A. Features of Change

1. Resistance usually accompanies the introduction of change.
2. Change is more comfortable when it is planned; unplanned change can lead to anxiety, resistance, and chaos.
3. Planned change occurs slowly.

B. Phases of Change (Lewin, 1947)

1. *Unfreezing*—Involves recognizing the need for change, and exposing and breaking down established myths and assumptions.
2. *Moving*—Involves giving up old habits and practices, and learning to use new methods and skills.
3. *Refreezing*—Involves instituting and reinforcing new attitudes, skills, knowledge, or behavior patterns.

C. Progression of Change

1. Change does *not* usually progress in a linear fashion from problem identification to solution.
2. The course of change is usually *not* smooth.

II. Changing to Restraint-Free Care

A. Groups to Target

1. Board of Directors/Owner(s)

The role of this group is to frame or approve broad organizational philosophy and policy. Members often view restraint use as the norm, and as a necessary but unfortunate component of care. Their concerns usually relate to (a) legal risk and practical response to behaviors that have often led to physical restraints, and (b) family response to change in practice and concern about "safety" of loved ones. A reframing of organizational philosophy to include individualized restraint-free care is essential if change is to occur.

2. Administration

Administrators oversee day-to-day operations, attend to needs of clients and staff, and promote fiscally responsible care. Their understanding of restraint-free care varies, depending on factors such as experience, education and values. Concerns of administrators are generally similar to those of boards of directors/owner(s). "Buy-in" from this group is also critical.

3. Medical Staff

Physicians oversee medical care and work with other health care providers to maximize functional abilities of clients. Legal risk is a major concern. Physicians may be unaware of the non-protective function and hazardous outcomes of physical restraint. They need to be educated about restraint-free care; current research, standards and regulations; and the existing philosophy of the facility.

4. Nursing Staff

Nursing staff provide and manage day-to-day care. Nurses are usually distressed about "tying people up." Many feel threatened by the idea of restraint-free care, however, because it raises questions about the quality of care that has traditionally been provided. Staff often view equipment such as geriatric chairs, with fixed tray tables, seat belts, and wrist ties/mitts as "supports," "safety devices," or "medical immobilization" rather than restraints. The truth of many myths associated with restraint use are assumed, for example, that:

a. Physical restraints eliminate serious injuries and minimize legal liability.
b. Minimal use of physical restraints adds excessively to staff overload and requires more staff.
c. No interventions exist for responding to behaviors frequently associated with restraint use.

As nurses, and the staff whom they supervise, are key to achieving changes in practice, educational and consultative efforts targeted at them are very important. Breaking down myths, and changing established ideas and habits, take time and consistent effort.

5. Clients

Clients are consumers of care. They express concerns related to invasion of privacy and fear of injury to self, as well as loss of choice. Clients often express concerns related to falls or injuries, or report previous experiences and observations with restraints. Most clients need more information on current standards of care and information on interventions supporting individualized approaches to care.

6. Family and friends

Family and friends of clients are consumers and advocates. They usually find restraint of their loved one to be repugnant; however, they often view restraint use as necessary to prevent falls, interference with treatment, or other behaviors, especially with cognitive impairment. They typically fear being responsible or guilty if the client suffers an injury when not restrained. Again, education and support of this group are needed if change is to occur.

B. Program Development and Implementation (see Appendix A)

1. Unfreezing Phase

a. Develop a philosophy of restraint-free care at the outset: Staff need to feel commitment and support "from the top." Copies of a facility's philosophy should be circulated and discussed throughout the institution.

b. Identify leaders responsible for implementation: Leader(s) must be committed and sincere about the program, and powerful enough to influence change. Leader(s) must have the credibility to deal with staff and the authority to facilitate change.
c. Set clear, achievable goals.
d. Provide fundamental educational program(s) regarding restraint-free care: Invite everyone, but ensure involvement of target groups (e.g., nursing, social service, medicine, psychiatry, rehabilitation therapies, families).
e. Facilitate open communication and dialogue regarding restraint-free care: Staff meetings, team conferences, and clinical rounds are appropriate forums.

2. Moving Phase

   a. Become aware of persons who are restrained.
   b. Determine the stated reason(s) for each restraint; investigate the precipitants of restraint.
   c. Eliminate restraints on the easiest cases first (in consultation with clients, family, and staff); success encourages staff to continue efforts with more difficult cases.
   d. Prohibit use of restraints once eliminated from a person or unit.
   e. Develop a "no restraint" protocol for new admissions.
   f. Establish a protocol for emergency response to specific behaviors (e.g., bed or chair alarm for fall risk).
   g. Create an evaluation or feedback system:

      (1) Monitor use of medications (e.g., Are psychoactive drugs used as "chemical restraints" a substitute for treatment of specific psychiatric problems?).
      (2) Monitor rates and circumstances of falls and injuries (e.g., Is the facility/unit rate of falls and injuries increased, decreased, unchanged, or different since the initiation of restraint free care?).
      (3) Circulate regular reports regarding progress toward goals (e.g., newsletters, memos).

   h. Provide continuing education for target groups, depending on needs.
   i. Celebrate efforts and successes.

3. Refreezing Phase

a. Develop and refine policies and procedures to reflect changes and new learning. (This is discussed in chapter 7.)
b. Adhere to policies and procedures in a consistent manner.

III. Clinical Models

A. Nursing Home

1. Formal education and unit-based clinical case consultation (Evans et al., 1997).

This approach to restraint-free care was implemented in a 180-bed religiously affiliated, non-profit facility as the intervention for a controlled clinical trial. Ten 30-to-45-minute educational sessions for all staff were provided twice during each shift over a 6-month period by a gerontologic nurse specialist (GNS). Sessions focused on consequences of physical restraint, making sense of behaviors, minimizing fall risk, preventing interference with medical treatment, and responding to behaviors. (Strumpf, Evans, Wagner, & Patterson, 1992). In addition, unit-based clinical case consultation was provided by the GNS for 12 hours/week over the same 6-month period. (Patterson, Strumpf, & Evans, 1995). Consultation efforts were directed mainly toward residents with behaviors that posed clinical challenges (e.g., cognitively impaired residents with multiple falls; residents with disturbing behaviors). Immediately following the 6-month intervention period, a 56% reduction in restraint use was noted, which was achieved without increases in staffing, psychoactive drug use, or serious fall-related injuries. A reduced level of restraint use was maintained at the facility at 3 months and 6 months after the intervention, although increases in restraint use began to occur once the GNS was no longer at the facility.

2. In-service training and multidisciplinary project team (Sundel, Garrett, & Horn, 1994).

This approach to restraint-free care was implemented in a 265-bed non-profit facility. One 90-minute inservice training session was provided for all employees. The session included: (a) a lecture on adverse effects of physical restraints; (b) a videotape entitled, "Untie the Elderly: The Change Makers," by the Kendal Corporation; (c) discussion of OBRA regulations related to restraint use; and (d) a sensitivity exercise, which involved restraining 10 employees for the entire 90-minute session to dramatize the physical and emotional experience of being restrained. The multidisciplinary project team consisted of representatives from nursing, social services, rehabilitation services, recreation therapy, and administration. The team was responsible for planning and supervising restraint reduction, activities that were eventually integrated into resident care planning meetings. Fourteen months after implementation of these initiatives, a significant reduction in the number of restrained residents was noted (from 67.5% to 36.7%, $p < 0.0001$), and more than twice as many employees supported restraint reduction (from 15.2% to 36.3%, $p < 0.0001$).

3. Statewide initiative (Rader, Semradek, McKenzie, & McMahon, 1992).

   This three-year demonstration project, funded by The Robert Wood Johnson Foundation, targeted all long-term-care facilities in Oregon. Leadership for the project was shared by a Coordinating Committee, Advisory Committee, and State Clinical Consultant for Nursing Home Practice.

   Members of the Coordinating Committee included: Representatives from the Oregon Association of Homes for the Aging, Oregon Health Care Association, and Senior and Disabled Services Division; a resident care manager; a consumer advocate; and the state clinical consultant for nursing home practice. The role of this committee was to coordinate restraint reduction efforts of providers, regulators, and consumers, and identify and resolve problems associated with implementation of OBRA guidelines.

   Members of the Advisory Committee included: representatives from the state ombudsman's office; physical, occupational, and speech therapy associations; Alzheimer's Disease and Related Disorders Association; state Mental Health Division; as well as geriatricians, geropsychiatrists, and other experts. The role of this committee was to provide liaison with interested groups and individuals in the state.

   Responsibilities of the State Clinical Consultant for Nursing Home Practice included: direction of the project, leadership of the Coordinating and Advisory Committees, provision of onsite consultation to selected nursing homes, and provision of telephone consultation to personnel at all levels. This role was tested during the project with the expectation that it would be continued as a state-funded position.

   Methods employed in this project included: (a) *education* in the form of train-the-trainer sessions for a mix of providers and regulators; (b) *consultation*, accomplished through the sharing of expertise within facilities, among facilities within regions, and at the state level; (c) *regulation*, which involved teaching and promotion of self-monitoring efforts; and (d) assistance with *problem-solving* and clarification of policy.

Following implementation of these initiatives, reduced restraint use was noted in most of Oregon's long-term-care facilities. Constant vigilance and reinforcement of individualized care was necessary, however, to prevent "backsliding" and substitution of one type of restraint for another.

4. The National Nursing Home Restraint Removal Project (Dunbar, Neufeld, White, & Libow, 1996).

   Funded by the Commonwealth Fund, The Jewish Home and Hospital for the Aged in New York City conducted a national demonstration to develop and evaluate safe and effective ways to replace physical restraints among nursing home residents. The goal was 5% restraint use or less in two years, both for facilities individually and in the aggregate.

   The project included 16 randomly selected facilities, 4 each from California, Michigan, New York, and North Carolina, with a total of 2,075 beds (Neufeld, Libow, Foley, & White, 1995). All had restraint rates above 30%, and the aggregate rate was 41% when the project began. Two years later, it had declined by 90%, to 4.05%. Serious injuries appeared to decline, the program was cost-effective, and the vast majority of staff and residents welcomed and approved it.

B. Hospital

1. Staff education and clinical case consultation (Strumpf & Evans, 1994–1998).

   This approach to restraint-free care is being implemented in a 600-bed urban teaching hospital as the intervention in a controlled clinical study of restraint reduction among hospitalized nursing home residents. A gerontologic nurse specialist (GNS) is available for all nursing staff providing care to nursing home residents admitted to participating hospital units. Using 1:1 consultation to hospital nurses and informal unit-based education (e.g., rounds, clinical conferences), individualized approaches to care and issues related to restraint use are resolved. Articles related to restraint-free care are posted regularly on the hospital's educational bulletin board, and a binder containing abbreviated information about restraints is available on all participating units.

Clinical case consultation is provided by the GNS, who conducts an assessment and develops an individualized plan of care with input from nursing home staff within 12 to 36 hours of a nursing home resident's admission to the hospital. The GNS visits the hospitalized resident daily to evaluate the resident's progress and recommend specific interventions for providing care without physical restraints and inappropriate psychoactive drugs. Contact with the resident's key caregivers in the hospital occurs daily during report, clinical rounds, or informal interaction initiated by the GNS. The GNS's individualized assessment, care plan, and progress notes are maintained at the resident's bedside, along with other standard hospital documentation forms; all consultation materials are faxed to the nursing home at the time of the resident's discharge from the hospital to facilitate continuity of care.

Outcomes and evaluation of the effectiveness of this approach should be available early in 1999.

2. Nursing task force: "Keeping People Healthy Initiatives" (Baldino, 1994).

   Restraint-free care is one of the objectives of this project, which is facilitated by advanced practice nurses in the Medical Nursing Department of a large urban teaching hospital. Through case consultation and forums for sharing "clinical narratives" (success stories), staff are assisted to develop creative strategies for disease prevention and health promotion. In cases involving older adults, advanced practice nurses are frequently consulted regarding approaches to individualized care and avoidance or reduction of restraint use.

3. System-wide geriatric planning committee (Bocchino, 1993; Bocchino et al., 1995).

   This approach to a system-wide restraint-free environment was implemented by a regional health care organization comprised of seven hospitals with a total of 1700 beds. The system-wide geriatric planning committee, which functions as a steering committee, is composed of the marketing manager, program development manager, and vice president of patient care for the hospital system. Membership on this committee is also accorded to representatives from various divisions, including physicians, social workers, marketing directors, home medical services directors, and nurses in the capacity of vice presidents of patient care, geriatric specialists, skilled nursing facility directors, and education directors. Initially, the committee engaged in a literature review, sought consultation from clinical and legal experts, and developed a position statement on restraint reduction, which was endorsed by the administrator of the hospital system, division presidents, division vice presidents of patient care, physicians, and the legal/risk management department. Subsequently, restraint reduction policies were created within each division, and pilot studies were initiated on selected units. One year after implementation of this approach, staff nurses were less likely to endorse restraint use, and a decline in the prevalence and duration of restraint use was observed system-wide.

IV. Summary

Restraint-free care involves commitment from key administrative leaders across disciplines and from all levels of staff. The process of change can be slow; a systematic method where individualized approaches to care are gradually introduced is most often successful. Education, available resources, and open communication also facilitate lasting change.

Bibliography

Baldino, J. (1994, December). Losing restraint. *HUPdate*, 14–15.

Blakeslee, J., Goldman, B., Papougenis, D., & Torell, C. (1991). Making the transition to restraint free care. *Journal of Gerontological Nursing, 17*(2), 4–8.

Bocchino, N. (1993, November). *A progress report: Changing restraint use in acute care.* Paper presented at the annual meeting of the American Geriatrics Society, New Orleans, LA.

Bocchino, N., Reed, C. R., Bradley, P. K., Cash, B., Downer, J., Rogers, P. D., & Tavolaro-Ryley, L. (1995). Effects of a restraint reduction pilot program in acute care. *The Gerontologist, 35*(Special Issue I), 168.

Colberg, A., Lynch, D., & Mavretish, B. (1991). Harnessing ideas to release restraints. *Geriatric Nursing, 12*(3), 133–134.

Dunbar, J. M., Neufeld, R. R., White, H. C., & Libow, L. S. (1996). Retrain, don't restrain: The educational intervention of the National Nursing Home Restraint Removal Project. *The Gerontologist, 36*(4), 539–542.

Ejaz, F. K., Folmar, S. J., Kaufman, M., Rose, M. S., & Goldman, B. (1994). Restraint reduction: Can it be achieved? *The Gerontologist, 34*, 694–699.

Evans, L. K., Strumpf, N. E., Allen-Taylor, S. L., Capezuti, E., Maislin, G., & Jacobsen, B. (1997). A clinical trial to reduce restraints in nursing homes. *Journal of the American Geriatrics Society, 45*(6), 675–681.

Hardin, S. B., Magee, R., Stratmann, D., Vinson, M. H., Owen, M., & Hyatt, E. C. (1994). Extended care and nursing home staff attitudes toward restraints: Moderately positive attitudes exist. *Journal of Gerontological Nursing, 20*(3), 23–31.

Harris, E. (1992). A journey to restraint free care. *Untie the Elderly, 4*(2), pp. 1, 6.

Jewish Home and Hospital for Aged. (1991). Retrain, don't restrain. Washington, DC: American Association of Homes and Services for the Aging.

Jewish Home and Hospital for Aged. (1991). Retrain, don't restrain. Washington, DC: The American Health Care Association.

Kapp, M. (1991, January). Reducing restraint use in nursing homes: The governing board's role. *Quality Review Bulletin*, pp. 22–25.

Kendal Corporation. (1996, December). Steps to restraint reduction. *Untie the Elderly, 8*(3), (Special Insert).

Lewin, K. (1947). Frontiers in group dynamics: Concept, method and reality in social science. *Human Relations, 1*, 5–42.

Mahoney, D. F. (1995). Analysis of restraint free nursing homes. *Image: Journal of Nursing Scholarship, 27*(20), 155–160.

Mion, L. C., & Mercurio, A. T. (1992). Methods to reduce restraints: Process, outcomes, and future directions. *Journal of Gerontological Nursing, 18*(11), 5–11.

Mount St. Mary's Nursing Home. (1990). *Going restraint free: Some suggestions*. Niagara Falls, NY: Hewner.

Neary, M., Kanski, G., Janelli, L., Scherer, Y., & North, N. (1991). Restraints as nurses' aides see them. *Geriatric Nursing, 12*(4), 191–192.

Neufeld, R. R., Libow, L. S., Foley, W., & White, H. (1995). Can physically restrained nursing home residents be untied safely? Intervention and evaluation design. *Journal of the American Geriatrics Society, 43*, 1264–1268.

Patterson, J. E., Strumpf, N. E., & Evans, L. K. (1995). Nursing consultation to reduce restraints in a nursing home. *Clinical Nurse Specialist, 9*(4), 231–235.

Rader, J., & Donius, M. (1991). Leveling off restraints. *Geriatric Nursing, 12*(2), 71–73.

Rader, J., Semradek, J., McKenzie, D., & McMahon, M. (1992). Restraint strategies: Reducing restraints in Oregon's long-term care facilities. *Journal of Gerontological Nursing, 18*(11), 49–56.

Schott-Baer, D., Lusis, S., & Beauregard, K. (1995). Use of restraints: Changes in nurses' attitudes. *Journal of Gerontological Nursing, 21*(2), 39–44.

Strumpf, N. E., Evans, L. K., Wagner, J., & Patterson, J. (1992). Reducing physical restraints: Developing an educational program. *Journal of Gerontological Nursing, 18*(11), 21–27.

Strumpf, N. E., & Evans, L. K. (1994–1998). *Maintaining restraint reduction in nursing homes* (1-RO1 AG08324). National Institute on Aging.

Sundel, M., Garrett, R. M., & Horn, R. D. (1994). Restraint reduction in a nursing home and its impact on employee attitudes. *Journal of the American Geriatrics Society, 42*, 381–387.

Werner, P., Cohen-Mansfield, J., Koroknay, V., & Braun, J. (1994). Reducing restraints: Impact on staff attitudes. *Journal of Gerontological Nursing, 20*(12), 19–24.

Williams, C. C., & Finch, C. (1997). Physical restraint: Not fit for woman, man, or beast. *Journal of the American Geriatrics Society, 45*, 773–775.

Yoshino, T. (1994). Restraint reduction program at Menorah Park. *Untie the Elderly, 6*(3), 1–3.

Appendix A

Restraint-Free Care: Program Development and Implementation

Unfreezing

- Develop a philosophy of restraint free care.
- Identify leaders responsible for implementation.
- Set clear, achievable goals.
- Provide fundamental education regarding restraint free care.
- Facilitate open communication and dialogue regarding restraint free care.

Moving

- Become aware of persons who are restrained.
- Determine the stated reason(s) for each restraint.
- Eliminate restraints on the easiest cases first.
- Prohibit use of restraints once they have been eliminated.
- Develop a "no restraint" protocol for new admissions.
- Establish a protocol for emergency response to specific behaviors.
- Create an evaluation or feedback system (track medication use, falls and injuries, and progress toward goals).
- Provide continuing education.
- Celebrate efforts and successes.

Refreezing

- Develop and refine policies and procedures to reflect changes.
- Adhere to policies and procedures in a consistent manner.

3

Making Sense of Behavior: Cornerstone of Individualized Care

Joanne Patterson Robinson and Pamela M. Zisselman

The Purpose of this Chapter is to:

1. Describe manifestations and meanings of behavioral phenomena.
2. Outline a method for assessing and evaluating behavior.
3. Emphasize the relationship between understanding behavior and individualizing care.

I. Perception of Behavior

Behavioral phenomena may be seen and understood by clinicians in numerous ways based upon their perceptions and clinical experiences. Once the clinician has perceived a behavior, he/she must investigate and make sense of it.

A. What is Perception?

1. Definition: Perception is a person's awareness and interpretation of stimuli. It is based on individual observation and understanding of the environment. (See Appendix A for an illustration of this concept.)

2. Mechanism:

   a. Stimuli in the environment seldom reach the sense organs (skin, eyes, ears, nose) alone; most compete with other stimuli for attention or become linked with numerous stimuli that are perceived in patterns.

      Example: The stimulus "snow" usually occurs as part of a pattern of stimuli that includes cold weather and gray clouds; however, the pattern is seen as a whole.

   b. Perception is the way individuals process information received by sense organs and attach meaning to this information; thus, individual perceptions of the same event can vary.

      Example: A person preparing to drive to work and a person about to start a vacation at a ski resort are likely to perceive the stimulus of "snow" differently. For one, it may evoke dismay, and for the other, joy.

B. What Influences Perception?

1. Condition of sensory organs.
2. Context of the situation.
3. Past experiences of the individual.
4. Health status.
5. Differential attention to various stimuli.

C. Key points about observing and describing behavior

1. It is critical that clinicians suspend their perception and attributions of behavior to really "see" what is happening. A clear description of behavior, without the perceiver's interpretations, is the first step toward making sense of behavior.
2. Behavior can be used to communicate needs, threats to self-esteem, a state of arousal, or severe anxiety. For example, sliding out of a chair may reflect the need to use the toilet, sense of hunger or thirst, feeling uncomfortable or weak, inability to maintain position, poor "fit" of the chair, or confusion.
3. Many commonly used terms do not clearly define the behavior of concern, e.g., "wandering," "sundowning," or "agitation." Use specific descriptors like "walking repeatedly into others' rooms" to begin analysis of behavior.

D. Clinical Implications

1. Because perception is highly individual, it is likely that clinician perceptions of a situation may be different from client perceptions. Exactly what the world looks like from the client's vantage point may be different from views held by care providers.
2. Many times, illusions created by the client's limited perspective of an unfamiliar environment and/or sensory limitations go unrecognized by clinicians.

   Example: An IV stand with a bag hanging from it, and positioned slightly outside the line of vision, may appear to the visually impaired as an unfamiliar person. A reasonable reaction to such a perception might be anxiety, presenting as restlessness or an attempt to escape by climbing out of bed. Thus, misperception of the environment as threatening may precipitate the behavior.

3. Perceptions and opinions about the meaning and cause of client behaviors vary among clinicians. It is thus important to validate client's perceptions of his/her situation, as well as to allow staff to share observations and thoughts about all possible reasons for behavior(s).

II. Clinical Evaluation of Behavior: Three Part Strategy (see Appendix B)

All behavior has meaning. It serves the older person in some manner, is goal directed and can be understood. Understanding the meaning of an individual's behavior requires a process of careful investigation and analysis.

A. Get to Know the Person (Rader & Tornquist, 1995)

1. Ask client about the behavior.
2. Obtain information from client and family about past life experiences, interests, pleasures, social and behavioral patterns, and activities or circumstances surrounding the present behavior.
3. Talk with care providers on other shifts and other members of the interdisciplinary team. Ask for observations, interpretations, and suggestions for responding to the behavior.
4. Review the health care record including:

   a. Preadmission/admission/transfer notes.
   b. Current plan of care.
   c. Progress notes.
   d. Physician orders.

e. Recent diagnostic tests.
f. Medication records.
g. Incident reports.
h. Consultation reports.

5. Perform or review assessment of overall health status.

a. Past and present health history.
b. Relevant findings from physical examination.
c. Current medications and treatments.
d. Recent diagnostic/laboratory studies.
e. Reversible conditions which may be related to or responsible for specific behaviors (e.g., infection, dehydration, drug toxicity, pain, depression).

6. Perform or review assessment of psychosocial status.

a. General appearance and behavior.
b. Psychological history.

1) Sources of pride.
2) Disappointments and regrets.
3) Coping strategies.
4) Education.
5) Work.
6) Recent role changes or losses.
7) Social interests.
8) Hobbies/activity involvement.
9) Relationships.
10) History of psychiatric illness.
11) Substance abuse.

c. Living situation.
d. Support systems.
e. Communication abilities/skills.
f. Financial status.
g. Spirituality.

1) Religious background.
2) Sources of meaning in life.
3) Hope for the future.
4) Understanding of death.
5) Needs related to expression of spirituality.

7. Perform or review assessment of functional status.

    a. Ambulation.
    b. Transfer.
    c. Bathing.
    d. Continence.
    e. Dressing.
    f. Feeding.

8. Perform or review assessment of mental status, considering the following points:

    a. Orientation: Impaired in both dementia and delirium.
    b. Attention and concentration: Always impaired in delirium.
    c. Psychomotor assessment: Certain drugs may cause psychomotor agitation or retardation in older adults. In addition, delirium and depression usually present with psychomotor disturbance.
    d. Speech: Assess receptive and expressive abilities in addition to the individual's rate and melody of speech.
    e. Thought form and content: Do statements by the individual make sense? Is s/he focused on certain ideas or certain concerns? For example, depressed individuals are often focused on perceived failings of themselves or their bodies. Perceptual disturbances such as illusions or visual hallucinations are often present in delirium.
    f. Memory: Impaired recent and remote memory can be present in depression, dementia or delirium.
    g. Judgment: Depressed individuals often forgo medical treatment that is otherwise acceptable when in a clearer frame of mind. Persons with dementia or delirium often have very limited comprehension of their illnesses and need for treatment.

B. Analyze the Context or Circumstances of the Behavior

This is as critical as documenting vital signs and weights. Visible behaviors and nonverbal communication are vital signs that are critical to providing individualized care for older adults without use of physical restraints or inappropriate psychoactive drugs.

1. When does the behavior occur? Exact dates and exact times help to target when intervention is needed and will be most effective.
2. What specific actions/interactions/reactions characterize the behavior?

3. Where does the behavior tend to occur? Look for patterns in the environment.
4. Who is present when the behavior occurs? What are others doing, and could this be upsetting or disturbing?
5. What could be happening internally (*inside the client*) to precipitate the behavior? What does the client say about the behavior? Could s/he be upset, lonely, in pain? Remember that behavior is a form of communication.
6. What could be happening externally (*outside the client*) to precipitate the behavior? Is the environment noisy, dark, shadowy, etc.? How do those present respond to the behavior? How does the client react to responses made by others?
7. What interventions help the client? If something helps, it may be a clue to what the behavior means. It is also important to document successful interventions that can be incorporated into the care plan.

C. Determine Meaning of the Behavior

Based on observed patterns, determine possible reasons for client perceptions of what is happening, what s/he is experiencing, what emotions are being communicated, and what the behavior means within his/her framework. Attempt to validate meaning of behavior with client and/or family member. Once behavior is understood from the client's perspective, interventions with positive effects on behavior can be tailored to individual needs.

An assessment tool for the clinical evaluation of behavior is the Behavior Log (see Appendix C).

1. Purpose: To facilitate consistent observation and documentation of behaviors so that pattern(s) and meaning can be determined.
2. Directions for use of Behavior Log (see Appendix D):

    a. Focus on one specific behavior at a time. Describe the behavior in clear, objective terms as it is observed (e.g., pulls tape off abdominal dressing, walks into others' rooms).
    b. Record specific observations of each episode of the designated behavior in relevant columns of the log.
    c. Continue to document each episode of behavior on the log until a pattern in its occurrence can be detected, e.g., Does behavior seem to occur at certain times of the day? Is there someone or something always present or happening in the environment when certain behaviors occur? Does behavior relate in any way to past life experiences (e.g., job, military, family life)?

d. Maintenance of the log for several episodes of the behavior will probably be necessary to detect patterns (see Appendix E for a Behavior Log in Progress).

III. Assess the Environment

A review of the following, in conjunction with the ongoing assessment of individuals, is also essential to understand impact of the system and the milieu on behavior. In many instances, the organizational, physical, and psychosocial environment will also require a process of change if resident and staff behaviors are to be modified and individualized restraint-free care achieved.

A. Organizational environment.

1. Philosophy.
2. Policy and procedures.
3. Staffing.
4. Routines.
5. Resource availability and allocation.

B. Physical environment.

1. Personalization and homelike features.
2. Noise levels.
3. Lighting.
4. Floor surfaces.
5. Design/suitability of equipment and furniture.
6. Visual cues.
7. Barriers to mobility.
8. Level of stimulation.
9. Space for privacy and socialization.
10. Safety and security.

C. Psychosocial environment.

1. Clothing.
2. Interaction patterns.
3. Activities.
4. Family support and education.
5. Counseling and consultation services.

IV. Outcome: Individualized care [see Appendix F]

Individualized approaches are key to understanding and caring for older adults (Fagan, Williams, & Burger, 1997; Happ, Williams, Strumpf, & Burger,

1996; Miller, 1994; Vollen, 1996). The goals of individualized care include promoting comfort and safe mobility, optimizing function and independence, and achieving the greatest possible quality of life. Such care requires clinicians to make sense of behavior rather than to control responses of clients. It is a philosophy of hopefulness. Reliance on physical and chemical restraint to control behavior is inconsistent with the practice of individualized care (see Appendix E). Essential components of individualized care include:

A. An interdisciplinary and person-centered approach.
B. Careful assessment of behavior and development of tailored interventions to meet specific needs.
C. Attention to the environmental milieu and overall system of care, especially features emphasizing a more normalized environment.

V. Summary

Making sense of behavior is based on the following assumptions: 1) All behavior has meaning; 2) an older person's needs are best met when behavior is understood; 3) systematic approaches are necessary to understand behavior; and 4) the philosophy of individualized care is the cornerstone to care of older adults and understanding behavioral phenomena.

Most behaviors that lead to restraint use are either indications of a change in health status or expressions of unmet needs, which, if understood, may be met appropriately. Chapters 4, 5, and 6 describe interventions for behavioral phenomena, fall risk, and treatment interference that are congruent with individualized, restraint-free care.

Bibliography

Athlin, E., Norberg, A., & Asplund, K. (1990). Caregivers' perceptions and interpretations of severely demented patients during feeding in a task assignment system. *Scandinavian Journal of Caring Sciences, 4*(4), 147–155.

Beck, C., Baldwin, B., Modlin, T., & Lewis, S. (1990). Caregivers' perception of aggressive behavior in cognitively impaired nursing home residents. *Journal of Neuroscience Nursing, 22*(3), 169–172.

Boettcher, E. G. (1983). Preventing violent behavior: An integrated theoretical model for nursing. *Perspectives in Psychiatric Care, 21*(2), 54–58.

Carveth, J. A. (1995). Perceived patient deviance and avoidance by nurses. *Nursing Research, 44*(3), 173–178.

Cohen-Mansfield, J., Billing, N., Lipson, S., Rosenthal, A. S., & Pawlson, L. G. (1990). Medical correlates of agitation in nursing home residents. *Gerontology, 36*, M150–M158.

Do you see what I see? (1994, February). Columbus, OH: *Highlights for children*, p. 2.

Evans, L. K. (1996). Knowing the patient: The route to individualized care. *Journal of Gerontological Nursing, 22*(3), 15–19.

Fagan, R. M., Williams, C. C., & Burger, S. G. (1997). *Meeting of Pioneers in Nursing Home Culture Change*. Lifespan: Rochester, NY. (Available by calling 716-454-3224, x 115).

Flaskerud, J. H. (1980). Perceptions of problematic behavior by Appalachians, mental health professionals, and lay non-Appalachians. *Nursing Research, 29*(3), 140–149.

Fletcher, K. (1990). Restraints should be a last resort. *RN, 53*(1), 52–56.

Folmar, S., & Wilson, H. (1989). Social behavior and physical restraint. *The Gerontologist, 29*, 650–653.

Gurland, B. J., Wilder, D. E., & Toner, J. A. (1987). A model for multidimensional evaluation of disturbed behavior in the elderly. In A. G. Awad, H. Durgst, & H. M. R. Meir (Eds.), *Disturbed behavior in the elderly*. New York: Pergamon Press.

Hallberg, I. R., & Norberg, A. (1990). Staffs' interpretation of the experience behind vocally disruptive behavior in severely demented patients and their feelings about it: An exploratory study. *International Journal of Aging and Human Development, 31*(4), 295–305.

Happ, M. B., Williams, C. C., Strumpf, N., & Burger, S. G. (1996). Individualized care for frail elders: theory and practice. *Journal of Gerontological Nursing, 22*(3), 6–14.

Lustbader, W. (1996). Tales from individualized care. *Journal of Gerontological Nursing, 22*(3), 43–46.

Miller, R. I. (1994). Managing disruptive responses to bathing by elderly residents. *Journal of Gerontological Nursing, 20*(11), 35–39.

Mion, L. C. (1996). Establishing alternatives to physical restraint in the acute care setting: a conceptual framework to assist nurses' decision making. *AACN Clinical Issues, 7*, 592–602.

Morris, J., Hawes, C., Murphy, K., Nonemaker, S., Phillips, C., Fries, B., & Mor, V. (1991). *Resident assessment instrument: Training manual and resource guide*. Natick, MA: Eliot Press.

Outlaw, F. H., & Lowery, B. J. (1994). An attributional study of seclusion and restraint of psychiatric patients. *Archives of Psychiatric Nursing, 8*(2), 69–77.

Podrasky, D. L., & Sexton, D. L. (1988). Nurses' reactions to difficult patients. *IMAGE: Journal of Nursing Scholarship, 20*(1), 16–21.

Rader, J., & Tornquist, E. M. (1995). *Individualized dementia care: Creative, compassionate approaches*. New York: Springer Publishing Co.

Schwartz, D. (1958). Uncooperative patients? *American Journal of Nursing, 58*, 75–77.

Scott, R. R., Bramble, K. J., & Goodyear, N. (1991). How knowledge and labeling of dementia affect nurses' expectations. *Journal of Gerontological Nursing, 17*(1), 21–24.

Shomaker, D. (1987). Problematic behavior and the Alzheimer patient; Retrospection as a method of understanding and counseling. *The Gerontologist, 27*(3), 370–375.

Strumpf, N. E., & Evans, L. K. (1994–1998). *Maintaining restraint reduction in nursing homes* (1 RO1 AGO 8324). Bethesda, MD: National Institute on Aging.

Strumpf, N. E., & Evans, L. K. (1988). Physical restraint of the hospitalized elderly: Perception of patients and nurses. *Nursing Research, 37*(3), 132–137.

Talerico, K., Capezuti, E., Evans, L., & Strumpf, N. (1995). Making sense of behavior: Individualized care based on needs of the older adult. *The Gerontologist, 35* (Special Issue 1), 128.

Vogelpohl, T. S., Beck, C. K., Heacock, P., & Mercer, S. O. (1996). "I can do it!" dressing: Promoting independence through individualized strategies. *Journal of Gerontological Nursing, 22*(3), 39–42.

Vollen, K. H. (1996). Coping with difficult resident behaviors takes time. *Journal of Gerontological Nursing, 22*(8), 22–26.

Wegner, D. E., & Vallacher, R. R. (1977). *Implicit psychology: An introduction to social cognition.* New York: Oxford University Press.

Williams, C. C. (1989). Liberation: Alternative to physical restraint. *The Gerontologist, 29*(5), 585–586.

Williams, C. C. (1990). Long term care and the human spirit. *Generations, XIV*(4), 25–28.

Appendix A
Perception Exercises

1. Note the different views of "reality" that are possible in the exercise below.

Do You See What I See?

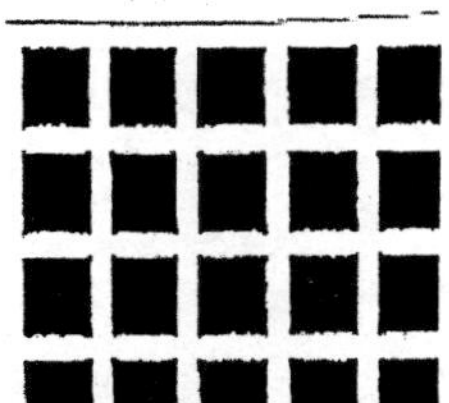

Do the white lines seem to have spots on them wherever they cross?

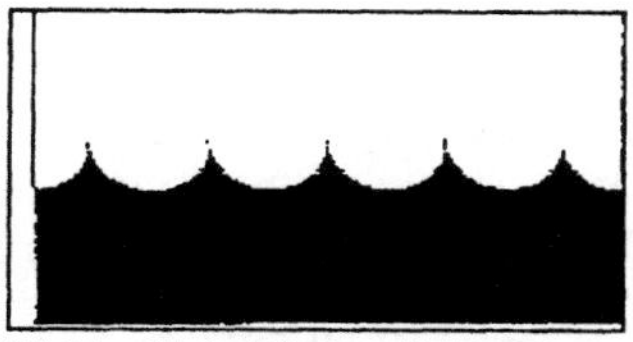

What does this look like to you? A curtain over a dark stage? Or maybe a row of circus tents?

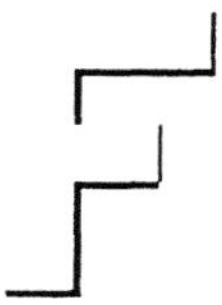

Are these just lines? Or do you see a letter of the alphabet?

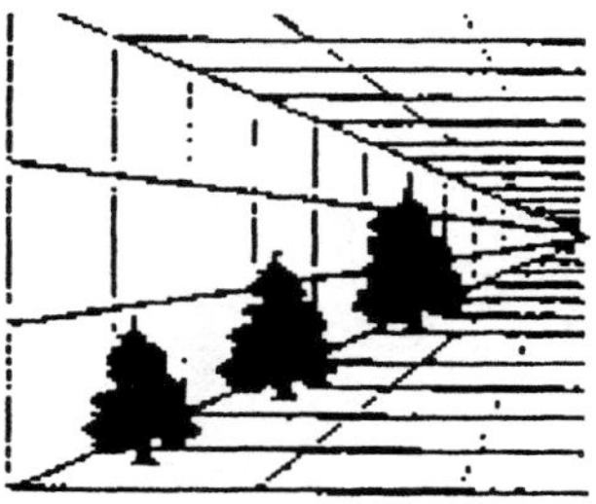

Which tree looks the tallest? Is it really tallest?

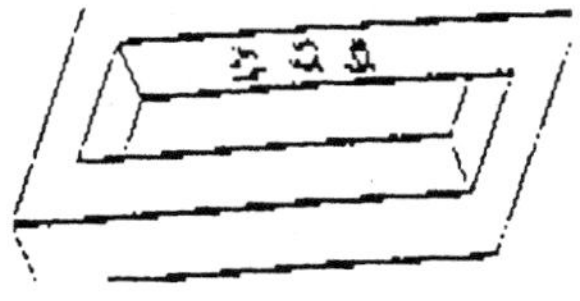

Are the ladybugs crawling on the inside? Or on the outside?

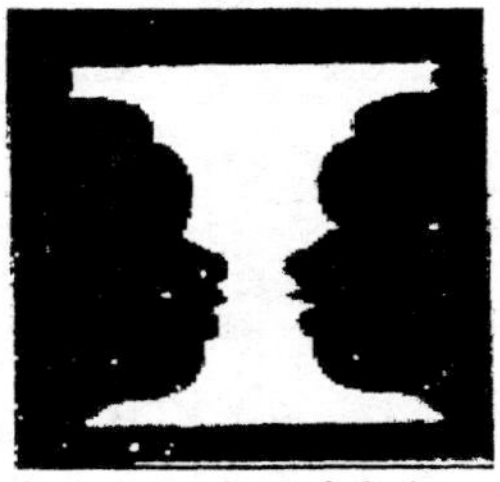

Is this a picture of a vase? Or do you see something else?

2. Distribute a piece of hard candy of the same flavor to several people and ask for a description of the candy. Several descriptions are likely (e.g., taste, texture, smell, color). This illustrates the point that individuals often attend to different attributes or aspects of the same object or experience.

Appendix B

Guidelines for the Clinical Evaluation of Behavior

1. *Get to know the person.*
   - Ask client about the behavior.
   - Obtain information from client and family about past life experiences, interests, pleasures, social and behavioral patterns, and activities or circumstances surrounding the present behavior.
   - Talk with care providers on other shifts and other members of the interdisciplinary team. Ask for observations, interpretations, and suggestions for responding to the behavior.
   - Review the resident's record, including:

     Preadmission/admission/transfer notes.
     Current plan of care.
     Progress notes.
     Physician orders.
     Recent diagnostic or other test procedures.
     Medication records.
     Incident reports.
     Consultation reports.

   - Perform or review assessments of:

     Overall health status.
     Psychosocial status.
     Functional status.
     Mental status.
     Environment.

2. *Analyze the context or circumstances of the behavior.*

- *WHEN* does the behavior occur?
- *WHAT* specific actions/interactions/reactions characterize the behavior?
- *WHERE* does the behavior occur?
- *WHO* is present when the behavior occurs?
- *WHAT* could be happening internally (*inside* the client) to precipitate the behavior?
- *WHAT* could be happening externally (*outside* the client) to precipitate the behavior?
- *WHAT* interventions help client?

3. *Determine meaning of the behavior using Behavior Log*:

   - Analyze patterns of behavior. For example:

     Does behavior seem to occur at certain times of the day?

     Is there someone or something always present or happening in the environment when certain behaviors occur?

     Does behavior relate in any way to the person's past life experiences (e.g., job, military, family life)?

   - Based on observed patterns, determine and validate possible reasons for client perceptions of what is happening, what s/he is experiencing, what emotions are being communicated, and what the behavior means.

REMEMBER: Making sense of behavior can be clinically challenging. Systematic approaches offer the best chance for discovering clues about the meaning of behavior and identifying responses that have positive effects on behavior.

Appendix C

Behavior Log

Specific Behavior: ____________________

Client's Name: ____________________ Room # ____________________

Date	Exact time	What hap-pened?	Where?	Who else was present?	What could be happening internally (*inside* client) to precipitate behavior?	What could be happening externally (*outside* client) to precipitate behavior?	What interventions help (could help) cli-ent?

Strumpf, N. E., & Evans, L. K. (1994–1998). *Maintaining restraint reduction in nursing homes* (1 RO1 AGO 8324). Bethesda, MD: National Institute on Aging.

Appendix D

Guidelines for Use of the Behavior Log

Purpose: To facilitate consistent observation and documentation of behaviors so that patterns(s) and meaning can be determined.

Directions for Use:

1. In the space next to the item labeled "Specific Behavior" record the behavior under observation (e.g., falls from bed, leaves unit, hits others, pulls at dressing).
2. Record the client's name and room number in the spaces provided.
3. Record specific observations for each episode of the designated behavior in relevant columns of the log:

   a. In Column 1, record the date of the observation of behavior.
   b. In Column 2, record the exact time when the behavior was observed.
   c. In Column 3, record exactly what behavior was observed (Example: fell from chair).
   d. In Column 4, record location where the episode occurred (Example: red chair in day room).
   e. In Column 5, note persons who were present and what they were doing (Example: Clients T. Jones & P. Smith; C.N.A. (Certified Nursing Assistant), F. Fox—talking with client T. Jones).
   f. In Column 6, describe what could be happening internally (*inside* the client) to precipitate the behavior (Example: Client stated she had to go to the bathroom urgently; had a diuretic at 9:00 AM).
   g. In Column 7, record what could be happening externally (*outside* the client) to precipitate the behavior (Example: No one available to take client to bathroom; floor recently polished).

h. In Column 8, describe what interventions helped (or could have helped) the client and resolve(d) the behavior (Example: Taken to bathroom every hour from 9:30 AM to 12:30 PM, then every other hour until bedtime; obtained new shoes with non-skid soles).

4. Continue observation and documentation of designated behaviors until a pattern(s) in occurrence can be detected (e.g., behavior seems to occur at specific times of the day; certain persons in the environment trigger a response; behavior corresponds with a lifetime habit of afternoon walks, etc.).
5. Maintenance of the log for several episodes of the behavior will probably be necessary to detect patterns. As interventions that alter the behavior are identified, these can be incorporated into the individualized care plan.

Appendix E

Example of Behavior Log in Progress

Specific Behavior: Frequent falls from chair
Client's Name: Sally Smith   Room # 123

Date	Exact time	What happened?	Where?	Who else was present?	What could be happening internally (*inside* client) to precipitate behavior?	What could be happening externally (*outside* client) to precipitate behavior?	What interventions help (could help) client?
1/10/98	11:30 AM	Fell from chair	Day room. Red chair by T.V.	2 clients: T. Jones & P. Smith	Stated she had to go to the bathroom urgently. Had a diuretic at 9:00 AM. Unsteady gait; needs 1 person assist for ambulation.	No one available to take to bathroom.	Taken to bathroom every hour from 9:30 AM to 12:30 PM, then every other hour until bedtime.

(continued)

Appendix E *(continued)*

Date	Exact time	What happened?	Where?	Who else was present?	What could be happening internally (*inside* client) to precipitate behavior?	What could be happening externally (*outside* client) to precipitate behavior?	What interventions help (could help) client?
1/12/98	10:30 AM	Fell from chair	Day room. Red chair by T.V.	CNA Fox talking with client T. Jones.	Stated she had to go to the bathroom urgently. Had a diuretic at 9:00 AM.	Floor had just been polished, wearing open backed slippers without a traction sole.	Obtained new shoes with non-skid soles.

Strumpf, N. E., & Evans, L. K. (1994–1998). Maintaining restraint reduction in nursing homes (1 RO1 AG0 8324). Bethesda, MD: National Institute on Aging.

Appendix F

Paradigm Shift Toward Individualized Care

HOPELESSNESS	vs.	HOPEFULNESS
↓		↓
CONTROL BEHAVIOR	vs.	**MAKE SENSE OF BEHAVIOR**
↓		↓
Goal of Care "Safety"	vs.	Goal of Care Safety plus: 1) Improve/Maintain Function and 2) Improve/Maintain Quality of Life
↓		↓
Physical Restraint Inappropriate Psychoactive Drug Use	vs.	Individualized Care

Adapted from: Talerico, K., Capezuti, E., Evans, L., & Strumpf, N. (1995). Making sense of behavior: Individualized care based on needs of the older adult. *The Gerontologist, 35* (Special Issue I), 128. [Paper presented at the Annual Meeting of Gerontological Society of America, November 1995].

4

Responding to Behavioral Phenomena

Pamela M. Zisselman and Lois K. Evans

The Purpose of this Chapter is to:

1. Understand a range of behavioral phenomena among cognitively impaired persons as a continuum of behaviors that are most often expressions of unmet needs or changes in health status.
2. Develop responses based on individualized care that eliminate use of restraints for behavioral phenomena.

I. Terminology and Description

In the literature, many terms are used to describe a range of behaviors often displayed by the older person with cognitive impairment. The terms include labels such as disturbing, challenging, problematic, disruptive and dysfunctional. Other terms used to describe behaviors are agitation, restlessness, wandering, and aggressiveness. Unfortunately, these terms do not define or identify the reasons for these behaviors but instead describe them in negative, dysfunctional or even pejorative terms. Such terminology may influence the reactions of staff who care for these older persons.

As discussed earlier, most behaviors have meaning and are caused by internal or external stimuli. An example is an older man with dementia, in great discomfort because of a fecal impaction and appearing agitated but nevertheless unable to verbalize the cause of his distress. As a result, he paces, yells, and cries throughout the unit. Once labeled as "agitated" by staff, and either sedated or restrained, it is unlikely the man will be further assessed or treated for the impaction. If the behavior is viewed by staff as an expression of an unmet need, however, the stage is set to complete a thorough assessment leading to appropriate interventions.

A. Impact of Behaviors

1. The effect of numerous behaviors is often distressing for all involved persons, in part because the behaviors seem to reflect discontent, frustration or suffering in the resident (Werner, Cohen-Mansfield, Braun, & Marx, 1989).
2. It may take a great deal of time and energy to respond to these behaviors.
3. Behavior perceived as disturbing by others often creates problems for the facility, family and person.
4. Behaviors viewed as disturbing by others often result in isolation for the person exhibiting them.
5. When large numbers of clients have behaviors viewed by staff as disturbing or challenging, the result may be increased staffing needs, along with greater staff burnout and turnover (Ryden, 1992).

B. Types of Behaviors

1. Psychomotor behaviors.

    a. Hiding objects; hoarding.
    b. Taking others' belongings.
    c. Inappropriate sexual behavior.
    d. Repetitive actions, e.g., removing clothing; unpacking/packing closets, drawers.
    e. Following others.
    f. Wandering:

        1) Wandering for a specific purpose, e.g., searching for someone.
        2) Non-directed.

    g. Physical aggression or assault, e.g., throwing objects, banging objects, kicking, hitting, or scratching others.
    h. Resisting treatment; refusing to follow directions.

2. Verbal behaviors.

   a. Repetitious speech patterns or "vocal tics."
   b. Yelling, calling out, talking loudly.
   c. Crying.
   d. Verbal abuse, e.g., constant complaints, insults, swearing, and anger with or without physical violence.

3. Psychological behaviors.

   a. Change in mood, e.g., dysphoria, withdrawal from environment, somatization, recurrent thoughts of death, suicidal ideation.
   b. Catastrophic reactions: Sudden changes in mood, often occurring in people with moderate cognitive impairment; associated with anger, agitation, pacing and/or physical aggression. Usually seems out of proportion to the precipitating event.

II. Assessment of Behaviors

A. It is the clinician's responsibility to investigate behavior (such as those listed above) and determine meaning.
B. General steps in the investigative process are covered in greater detail in chapter 3.

III. Triggers, Precipitators, or Contributing Factors

Identifying and understanding the factors underlying behavior requires time, but is well worth the effort in terms of outcomes for staff and patients/residents. Possible explanations for varying and often complex behaviors include physiological, environmental, or psychosocial factors.

A. Physiological Factors

1. Delirium.
2. Depression.
3. Dementia.

   Note: Clinicians should review the American Psychiatric Association's *Diagnostic and Statistical Manual of Mental Disorders* (1994) for criteria for evaluating and establishing the presence of delirium, depression, and dementia.

4. Physical discomfort may trigger numerous behaviors. Often internal noxious stimuli lead to an external response such as yelling or hitting. Some examples include:

a. Pain.
b. Feeling uncomfortably hot or cold.
c. Thirst.
d. Hunger.
e. Incontinence.
f. Constipation.
g. Urinary retention.
h. Fatigue.
i. Sleep deprivation.

B. Environmental Factors

1. Overstimulation.
2. Excessive or loud noise.
3. Understimulation.
4. Poor control of room temperature.
5. Care provider factors:

   a. Limited opportunities for relationships between care provider and older person, including frequent rotation of assignments.
   b. Rigid, task-oriented care versus person-oriented care.
   c. Inadequate training in relationship-centered, individualized care for nursing assistants and other care providers.

C. Psychosocial Factors

1. Invasion of personal space is the most common trigger of behavior perceived as difficult by clinicians and staff (Miller, 1994; Ryden & Feldt, 1992). It most often occurs during activities of daily living, specifically bathing and dressing. For example, in a nursing home, personal hygiene measures are often performed according to institutional routine, rather than longstanding personal habits and preferences. The public nature of shower rooms, and bathing by strangers, may insult an older person's sense of privacy and dignity.
2. Loss of control is often intensified, e.g., a nursing home resident may be offered no choice of bathing time.
3. Reduced sense of personal identity occurs when individual needs and preferences are subordinated to institutional efficiencies.
4. Feeling unsafe and insecure is common, especially when moving to a new room and meeting a new roommate; experiencing new routines; and meeting new staff.

IV. Strategies for Responding to Behavior

Care providers must understand and respond to underlying precipitants of behavior. Behaviors occur along a continuum: Unmet needs can escalate and become difficult to diagnose and treat. Ideally, the goal of care is to identify and treat unmet needs or changes in health status, thus preventing or minimizing behavioral phenomena. Examples of specific interventions (to be used depending on assessment of the behavior), follow:

A. Strategies for Responding to Physiological and/or Psychological Manifestations of Behavior:

1. Identify and treat etiologies of delirium, e.g.,

   a. Treat infection, hypoxia, and/or other precipitating agents.
   b. Reduce or eliminate exacerbating or inappropriate medications.
   c. Consider a short-term, low dose neuroleptic appropriate for specific target symptoms.

2. Treat depression, e.g.,

   a. Obtain evaluation and consider administration of an antidepressant.
   b. Increase socialization, pleasant activities, exercise.
   c. Provide supportive psychotherapy.
   d. Evaluate for electroshock therapy (ECT).

3. Treat discomfort, e.g.,

   a. Offer pain medication.
   b. Offer fluids.
   c. Offer food.
   d. Offer/remove sweater or blankets.
   e. Maintain a regular schedule and assistance for use of toilet, commode, urinal, bed pan.
   f. Manage and eliminate constipation/incontinence.
   g. Reposition, use supportive seating.

B. Strategies Employing Environmental Modifications in Response to Specific Behaviors:

1. Provide, as appropriate, an optimal level of stimulation, e.g.,

   a. Decrease traffic through unit.
   b. Decrease excess noise from speaker system, radio and television.
   c. Adjust for softer lighting.

2. Increase daytime stimulation, including psychosocial interaction, for persons experiencing "sundown syndrome." Other responses which may reduce sundowning include:

    a. Use night lights.
    b. Move person closer to nurse's station.
    c. Have night activities available, e.g., snacks, activity cart.
    d. Reduce sleep disturbing conditions.

3. Allow adequate and protected space, or other redesign specific for safe ambulation, e.g.,

    a. Sheltered courts, gardens, lounges.
    b. Irregular spaces and circular loops that suggest exploration rather than a sense of containment.
    c. Cues (signs) which compensate for memory loss. Reinforce the location of washroom, lounge, dining room, etc., by placing a drawing or photo of the activity which occurs in the room on the door; place an old photo of the person on the door of his/her room.
    d. Camouflage on doors and exits, including such methods as:

        1. Securing a cloth panel over door and covering door knob.
        2. Placing a planter or screen in front of door.
        3. Incorporating door in a wall mural.
        4. Painting door knob the same color as the door.

    e. Barriers to exit at doors, e.g., specialized locks.
    f. Special monitoring devices and alarms.

    Note: An organized retrieval system should be in place, including a facility-wide plan of response when a person is missing.

4. Provide as many home-like, normalized, and familiar features throughout the environment as possible.
5. Remove all physical restraints from the unit.

C. Strategies Employing Activities in Response to Specific Behaviors:

Individual and small group activities geared to the person's cognitive skills and interests may prevent or attenuate behaviors. Examples of such activities include:

1. Pet therapy.
2. Music group, with or without dancing.

3. Foot or hand massage.
4. Reminiscing, e.g., travel slides, pictures, familiar objects from the past.
5. Playing musical instruments, sing-alongs.
6. Folding linen or engaging in other repetitive but useful activities or movements.
7. Tossing a beach ball in a circle or other group activities.
8. Exercise, including walking and stretching.
9. Attending to flowers, plants, pets.
10. Group painting.
11. Food preparation (with appropriate supervision).
12. Simple and appropriate cleaning tasks.
13. Involvement in rounds with nursing staff if wandering or sleeplessness occurs at night.

D. Strategies Employing Psychosocial Responses to Specific Behaviors:

See the Matrix of Behaviors and Interventions, chapter 7, Appendix A, for further suggestions.

V. Medication Management

Medications are a potentially useful therapeutic modality in the care of cognitively impaired older persons. A careful investigation of behavior must be undertaken before any administration of psychoactive drugs as a treatment for behavioral phenomena occurs. Pharmacotherapy can be used effectively in conjunction with other psychosocial and/or environmental interventions. Individualized care is more than administration of a drug. Consultation by a geriatric psychiatrist and/or geropsychiatric nurse specialist is advised prior to initiating pharmacotherapy.

Various classes of medications for alleviating behavioral symptoms associated with dementia have been studied. Recently released psychoactive medications which may have more favorable side-effect profiles for elderly persons are currently being investigated.

A. Antipsychotic Medications

Antipsychotic drugs have some utility in the treatment of psychosis as well as alleviating certain "agitated" behaviors.

1. Examples of drugs include:

a. Haloperidol.
b. Risperidone.

   c. Thiothixene.
   d. Perphenazine.

2. Side effects: Sedation, drug-induced Parkinsonian syndrome, orthostatic hypotension, and tardive dyskinesia.
3. Dosing:

Drug	*Starting dose*	*Maximum dose*
Haloperidol	.25 mg/day	2 mg/day
Risperidone	.25 mg/day	2 mg/day
Thiothixene	2 mg/day	7 mg/day
Perphenazine	2 mg/day	8 mg/day

B. Antidepressant Medications

These drugs are useful with behaviors that may be mediated by an underlying depression.

1. Examples of drugs include:

   a. Sertraline.
   b. Paroxetine.
   c. Trazadone. Note: Not usually used as an antidepressant, but used to alleviate behaviors.

2. Side effects:

   a. Sertraline and Paroxetine: Excitation and gastrointestinal upset.
   b. Trazadone: Sedation and hypotension.

3. Dosing:

Drug	*Starting dose*	*Maximum dose*
Sertraline	25 mg/day	150 mg/day
Paroxetine	10 mg/day	40 mg/day
Trazadone	25 mg/day	150 mg/day

C. Mood Stabilizers

This class of drugs may also be beneficial with older, cognitively impaired persons with labile moods and behaviors that have been unresponsive to other measures.

1. Examples of drugs include:

a. Valproic Acid.
b. Carbamazepine.
c. Lithium Carbonate.

2. Side effects:

a. Valproic Acid and Carbamazepine: Hepatotoxicity, sedation, aplastic anemia, gastrointestinal upset, Stevens-Johnson syndrome (carbamazepine only).
b. Lithium Carbonate: Drowsiness, tremor, hypothyroidism, polyuria, polydipsia.

3. Dosing:

Drug	*Starting dose*	*Therapeutic blood level*
Valproic Acid	125 mg/bid	40–120 mcg/ml
Carbamazepine	50 mg/bid	5–10 mcg/ml
Lithium Carbonate	150 mg/day	0.3–1.0 mEq/liter

V. Summary

The philosophy of individualized care assumes that each person is unique and has a pre-existing lifetime of preferences and routines. Many cognitively impaired older adults display behaviors that reflect an attempt to maintain continuity, yet may pose unique challenges for clinicians. It is the role of care providers to investigate the behavior, determine its meaning, and develop strategies meeting expressed needs, thus responding positively to the current behavior and minimizing future episodes. Key points to remember are that:

A. All behaviors have meaning. Behaviors serve the person in some manner and need to be understood through a careful process of investigation.
B. Investigation includes obtaining a life history, performing a physical examination, and assessing behavior patterns (see chapter 3).
C. Many behaviors may be related to delirium, depression, dementia, and other physical and psychological discomforts.
D. Environmental and psychosocial factors may trigger a wide range of behaviors, including what appear to care providers as aggression, agitation, restlessness, unsafe mobility, etc.
E. Interventions include individualizing care and modifying the environment to fit personal needs and preferences. Selected psychoactive drugs may also be an appropriate treatment for specific behaviors, but should only be

initiated following consultation. Any psychoactive drug use requires ongoing follow-up and evaluation.

Bibliography

American Psychiatric Association. (1994). *Diagnostic and Statistical Manual of Mental Disorders, Fourth Edition*. Washington, DC: Author.

Bridges-Parlet, S., Knopman, D., & Thompson, T. (1994). A descriptive study of physically aggressive behavior in dementia by direct observation. *Journal of the American Geriatrics Society*, *42*, 192–197.

Burgio, L., Scilley, K., Hardin, J., Hsu, C., & Yaney, J. (1996). Environmental "white noise": An intervention for verbally agitated nursing home residents. *Journal of Gerontology: Psychological Sciences, 51*, 364–373.

Cohen-Mansfield, J., & Werner, P. (1998). The effects of an enhanced environment on nursing home residents who pace. *The Gerontologist, 38*(2), 199–208.

Evans, L., Strumpf, N., & Williams, C. (1991). Redefining a standard of care for frail older people: Alternatives to routine physical restraint. In P. Katz, R. Kane, & M. Mezey (Eds.), *Advances in Long Term Care, I*. New York: Springer Publishing Co., 81–108.

Everitt, D., Fields, D., Sounerai, S., & Avorn, J. (1991). Resident behavior and staff distress in the nursing home. *Journal of the American Geriatrics Society, 39*, 729–798.

Happ, M. B., Williams, C. C., Strumpf, N., & Burger, S. G. (1996). Individualized care for frail elders: Theory and practice. *Journal of Gerontological Nursing, 22*(3), 6–14.

Holmberg, S. K. (1997). A walking program for wanderers: Volunteer training and development of an evening walker's group. *Geriatric Nursing, 18*, 160–165.

Kovach, C. R., & Meyer-Arnold, E. A. (1997). Preventing agitated behaviors during bath time. *Geriatric Nursing, 18*, 112–114.

Miller, C. A. (1997). Behavior-modifying medications for mentally frail elders. *Geriatric Nursing, 18*, 89–90.

Miller, R. I. (1994). Managing disruptive responses to bathing by elderly residents. *Journal of Gerontological Nursing, 20*(11), 35–39.

Namazi, K., Rosner, T., & Calkins, M. (1989). Visual barriers to prevent ambulatory Alzheimer's patients from exiting an emergency door. *The Gerontologist, 29*, 699–702.

Rader, J. (1991). Modifying the environment to decrease use of restraints. *Journal of Gerontological Nursing, 17*(2), 9–13.

Rantz, M. J., & McShane, R. E. (1995). Nursing interventions for chronically confused nursing home residents. *Geriatric Nursing*, *16*, 22–27.

Ryden, M. B., & Feldt, K. S. (1992). Goal directed care: Caring for aggressive nursing home residents with dementia. *Journal of Gerontological Nursing, 18*(11), 35–41.

Simon, L., Jewell, N., & Brokel, J. (1997). Management of acute delirium in hospitalized elderly: A process improvement project. *Geriatric Nursing, 18*, 150–154.

Vollen, K. H. (1996). Coping with difficult resident behaviors takes time. *Journal of Gerontological Nursing, 22*(8), 22–26.

Werner, P., Cohen-Mansfield, J., Braun, J., & Marx, M. (1989). Physical restraints and agitation in nursing home residents. *Journal of the American Geriatrics Society, 37*, 1122–1126.

5

Assessment of Fall Risk and Prevention of Injurious Falls

Pamela M. Zisselman and Joanne Patterson Robinson

The Purpose of this Chapter is to:

1. Enhance knowledge of prevalence, pattern, and outcome of falls in older persons.
2. List intrinsic and extrinsic risk factors related to falls in older persons.
3. Identify components of a fall risk assessment.
4. Develop individualized approaches for preventing falls and serious injuries.
5. Identify the hazards of side rails and assess the need for their use.

I. Overview of the Problem

The goal of a fall prevention program is to minimize older adults' risk of falling and sustaining injuries without compromising mobility or functional independence. In an older adult, the probability of a fall increases as a function of the number of fall risk factors present. Thus, an individualized intervention designed to identify and eliminate modifiable fall risk factors is the most promising strategy (Tinetti, Baker, McAvay, et al., 1994; Tinetti, Doucette, & Clause, 1995).

A. Definition of a Fall: An event that results in a person coming to rest inadvertently on the ground or other lower level.

B. Prevalence

1. Nursing homes: While fall rates vary from one facility to the next, it is estimated that approximately 40% to 50% of nursing home residents fall annually.
2. Community settings: About 30% of community-dwelling elderly fall one or more times each year. Of those who report falling, about half report more than one fall during the year.
3. Hospitals: Falls account for 70% to 80% of in-patient incidents in acute care hospitals; incidents occur at a rate of 18 to 24 per 10,000 patient days; the majority of patients in acute care hospitals are elderly.

C. Patterns

1. Time: Falls occur most often during the busiest time of day (i.e., daytime), presumably consistent with increased levels of client activity.
2. Place: Older adults commonly fall in bathrooms and bedrooms.
3. Activity: Falls most often occur incidental to usual activities of daily living such as walking and transferring to or from bed, wheelchair/ chair, toilet/commode.
4. Person:

   a. Age—The risk of falling increases with age and rises more steeply after age 75.
   b. Gender—Falling is more frequent among females than males until age 85, when the frequency of falling is nearly equal among males and females.
   c. Race—Studies indicate a slightly higher rate of falls among Whites than among Blacks.
   d. Functional status—Falling is more frequent among the physically and cognitively impaired.

D. Outcomes of Falls

1. Injury is a leading cause of death among people over the age of 65; of these injuries, most are related to falls.
2. Most falls, however, do not result in *serious* injury:

   a. Only 3% to 5% of falls by older persons (age 65+), whether living in the community or in an institution, result in a fracture; about 1% result in hip fracture. In persons 85 years of age and older, 10% of falls result in hip fractures or other serious injuries.

b. Approximately 5% to 10% of falls result in severe soft tissue injuries; e.g., hematoma, sprains, joint dislocations. Devastating injuries, including subdural hematomas and cervical fractures, are rare.

3. Falls affect the elderly by impairing confidence and creating a sense of insecurity and fear, often resulting in self-imposed limitations in mobility and dependence upon others.

II. Risk Factors for Falls in the Elderly (see Appendix A)

A. Intrinsic Factors. There is a direct relationship between number of intrinsic risk factors and risk of falling. Intrinsic factors generally include medical conditions.

1. Acute and Chronic Illnesses.

a. Metabolic abnormalities.

1. Hyponatremia/hypovolemia.
2. Hypoglycemia.
3. Dehydration.

b. Arrhythmias may cause a syncopal episode.
c. Orthostatic hypotension.
d. Vasovagal episodes (fainting) may be caused by:

1. Defecation.
2. Valsalva.
3. Stress.

e. Sensory deficits/corrective devices.

1. Visual changes or impairments related to cataracts, macular degeneration, glaucoma, or use of bi- or tri-focals (especially on stairs).
2. Distortions and misperceptions related to hearing loss or vestibular dysfunction.
3. Vertigo and dizziness related to labyrinth disorders.

2. Dementia leading to alterations in judgment.
3. Incontinence (actual or potential).
4. Medications.

a. Anesthetics.
b. Antipsychotics.
c. Antihistamines.
d. Anticonvulsants.
e. Benzodiazepines, including sedative-hypnotics.
f. Cardiac drugs (e.g., diuretics, antihypertensives, calcium channel blockers).
g. Hypoglycemics.
h. Narcotics.
i. Use of multiple medications is also an intrinsic risk factor.

5. Musculoskeletal Risk Factors.

a. Normal age-related changes: bone degeneration (osteoporosis), kyphosis, and diminished muscle mass, muscle strength, joint resiliency, and ligament elasticity.
b. Prolonged bed rest results in loss of muscle strength and mass, and bone loss.
c. Degenerative joint diseases (osteoarthritis) causes painful joints, swelling, stiffness and decreased mobility.
d. Foot problems (e.g., deformities, bunions).

6. Neurologic Risk Factors.

a. Normal age-related changes: Delayed reaction time, diminished sensation in lower extremities, altered body sway, and changes in gait.
b. Transient ischemic attack (TIA).
c. Seizure.
d. Stroke.
e. Parkinson's disease.
f. Peripheral neuropathies (loss of pain, touch, position sense).

B. Extrinsic Risk Factors

1. Situational.

a. Poorly maintained or improperly used walking aids and other assistive devices.
b. Relocation to an unfamiliar environment.
c. Hurrying.
d. Performance of unusual activities.
e. Restraint reduction (may be associated with greater risk of noninjurious falls).

2. Environmental.

   a. Ground surfaces.

      1) Scatter rugs.
      2) Loose carpeting (e.g., torn, untaped, untacked).
      3) Slippery floors (wet or waxed).
      4) Obstructed pathways (e.g., cords, wires, low-lying objects).
      5) Door steps and uneven stairs: Stairs in general create a challenge because of diminished perceptions of height, depth, and surface edges.
      6) "Busy" floor patterns.
      7) Surface irregularities.

   b. Furniture.

      1) Clutter.
      2) Unstable furniture.
      3) Low furniture (e.g., coffee tables).
      4) Low chairs without armrests or seat backs.
      5) High beds.
      6) Cabinets which are either too high or too low.
      7) Absence of railings (hallways, stairs).

   c. Lighting.

      1) Glare from unshielded windows or lamps or highly polished floors.
      2) Dim lighting with dark walls.
      3) Absence of night lights.

   d. Bathroom.

      1) Low toilet seats and/or absence of slip-resistant strips, secure grab bars.
      2) Absence of non-slip surfaces or assistive devices in bathtub.
      3) Inappropriate placement of grab bars or assistive devices.

   e. Other.

      1) Ill-fitting clothing.
      2) Improper shoes (e.g., high-heeled, poorly fitted).
      3) Presence of tubes, catheters, etc.

III. Fall-Risk Assessment (see Appendix B)

A. Goal: Identify intrinsic and extrinsic risk factors.
B. History: Review previous fall situation(s) for intrinsic factors (e.g., hypotension due to dehydration), associated activities (e.g., trips to the bathroom), and extrinsic factors (e.g., wet floor) associated with fall risk.
C. Medication Review

1. Note recent changes in medication(s).
2. Check use of anesthetic, antidepressant, antihistamine, antipsychotic, anticonvulsant, benzodiazepine, cardiac, cathartic, hypoglycemic, or narcotic drugs.

D. Physical Exam

A focused physical exam is necessary to assess for presence of medical conditions which would place an older person at increased risk of falls.

1. Postural vital signs.
2. Mental status.

    a. Memory (recent and remote).
    b. Depression screen.

3. Sensory.

    a. Vision (Snellen chart).
    b. Hearing (Whisper test).

4. Neurological.

    a. Muscle tone.
    b. Presence of tremors.
    c. Motor strength (upper and lower extremities).
    d. Proprioception.

5. Musculoskeletal.

    a. Range of motion.
    b. Presence of joint deformities.
    c. Condition of feet.

6. Mobility—"Get-Up and Go Go Test" (Rader & Tornquist, 1995).

The Get Up and Go Go Test is a variation of the Get Up and Go Test developed by Mathias, Nayak, and Isaacs (1986). The second "Go" represents the addition of observations related to use of the toilet.

a. To conduct the Go Go test, observe performance in the following sequence of activities:

1) Sitting and standing from a chair.
2) Turning (360°) while standing.
3) Walking or wheeling to the bathroom or toilet.
4) Getting onto and using the toilet (includes observation of clothing management and post-elimination hygiene).
5) Getting off the toilet and sitting in a wheelchair, if used.
6) Walking or wheeling from the toilet or bathroom to the bed.
7) Getting into and out of bed.

b. Note evidence of the following risk factors:

1) A wide base of support.
2) Loss of balance while standing.
3) Balance problems when walking.
4) Decreased coordination.
5) Lurching, swaying, or sloping gait.
6) A need to hold on or change gait pattern when walking through a doorway.
7) Instability when making turn.
8) Improper use of assistive devices (e.g., walker, cane, wheelchair, furniture).
9) Difficulty with transfer to or from chair, toilet, or bed without help (e.g., use of furniture or other person(s) for assistance).

E. Laboratory Evaluation—Based on findings from history and physical exam, the following tests may be indicated:

1. CBC (to rule out anemia).
2. Electrolytes.
3. ECG (to rule out arrhythmia).
4. Drug levels.
5. CT or MRI of head.

Completion of a Fall-Risk Assessment in profiling the fall-prone older person (see Appendix C). Once a person is identified as high risk, any one or more of the following interventions may be appropriate.

IV. Interventions Directed Toward Intrinsic Risk Factors

A. Interventions aimed at ameliorating acute and chronic illnesses (Tinetti & Speechly, 1989).

1. Acute and chronic illness.

a. Diagnose and treat specific illness; e.g., pneumonia, urinary tract infection, delirium, dehydration.
b. Sensory function—optimizing vision and hearing are an integral part of a fall prevention program.

(1) Hearing.

(a) Perform audiologic evaluation.
(b) Remove cerumen.
(c) Use hearing aid as appropriate.
(d) Check batteries of hearing aids every two weeks.

(2) Vision.

(a) Diagnose and treat ophthalmologic problems as clinically indicated; e.g., cataracts, glaucoma. If treated, these conditions may improve and lower fall risk.
(b) Maintain up-to-date eyeglass prescription.
(c) Keep glasses clean.
(d) Use low vision aids and rehabilitative programs.
(e) Employ environmental adaptions, e.g., good lighting, clutter-free pathways, bright colored tape on steps.

2. Postural hypotension.

a. Avoid causative drugs, e.g., tricyclic antidepressants and diuretics.
b. Rehydrate and maintain hydration (1500–2000 cc/24 hours unless otherwise restricted).
c. Wear compression stockings as indicated.
d. Educate about methods of getting out of bed or chair:

(1) Rise slowly.
(2) Dorsiflex feet in bed.
(3) Count to thirty.
(4) Use handgrip in bed.

3. Dementia.

a. Educate family about falls.
b. Have family or companion accompany patient through admission process.
c. Provide a room assignment near nurses' station.
d. Avoid sedating or centrally acting drugs.
e. Supervise exercise and ambulation.
f. Assure a safe environment.
g. Offer structured activities, e.g., music, reminiscence.
h. Maintain consistent daily routine.
i. Eliminate excessive noise.

4. Incontinence (actual or potential).

a. Diagnose etiology.
b. Treat urinary tract infection.
c. Maintain timed voiding schedule.
d. Place handrail between bed and bathroom.
e. Keep commode near bedside.
f. Use nonskid strips at bedside, commode, and floor of bathroom, as well as nonslip, washable mat at commode.
g. Provide adequate lighting in bathroom and bedroom.
h. Provide easily manipulated clothing, e.g., velcro closures and elastic waistbands.

5. Medications.

Reduction of inappropriate medications may prevent falls in older adults. Interventions include:

a. Assessment of drug actions, interactions and side effects.
b. Determine the lowest effective dose.
c. Attempt to taper and eliminate medications when feasible.
d. Select short-acting medications.
e. Avoid drugs which put older adults at risk for falls, including sedatives, phenothiazines and tricyclic antidepressants.
f. Start at a low dose and increase slowly when initiating a new medication.

B. Interventions for Gait, Mobility, and Balance

Research demonstrates that older adults who exercise regularly have a reduced risk of falls (Lord, Ward, Williams & Strudwick, 1995; Province, Hadley, Hornbrook, et al., 1995). Older adults with neurologic problems such as Parkinson's disease, stroke and peripheral neuropathies may benefit from a regular physical therapy program.

1. Benefits of regular exercise include:

    a. Increased aerobic capacity.
    b. Improved gait and gait velocity.
    c. Increased skeletal muscle strength.
    d. Improved postural sway.
    e. Improved ability to climb stairs.
    f. Reduced falls.

2. Physical activity programs promote rehabilitative care rather than custodial care. Ideal exercise programs should be:

    a. Multidisciplinary (nursing, occupational therapy, physical therapy, and medicine).
    b. Individualized so that all older adults may participate.
    c. Developed through involvement of all staff.
    d. Motivational and include incentive programs and awards (e.g., monthly walking distance poster, awards program).
    e. Socially oriented, e.g., walking clubs.
    f. Stimulating, e.g., by offering a variety of exercises, including aerobic activity, flexibility training, balance and resistance training, and Tai Chi.

V. Interventions Directed Toward Extrinsic Factors

B. Environmental Interventions—Fall prevention programs include environmental adaptations for reducing an older person's fall risk and maintaining mobility and function (Donius, 1995; Grisso, Capezuti, & Schwartz, 1996; Tinetti & Speechly, 1989).

1. Environmental modifications applicable to bedroom, bathroom, and hallway:

    a. Wax-free floors, or low buff on waxed floors, using anti-skid acrylic wax.
    b. Adhesive strips on floor at bedside and commode.
    c. Night lights.
    d. Nonskid mats and strips for bathtub and shower.
    e. Object-free pathways.
    f. Electronic warning devices, e.g., bed monitors.

g. Handrails between bathroom and bed.
h. Rest stops, e.g., a chair midway between bed and bathroom or in hallway between bedroom and activity rooms.

2. Modifications in Beds and Chairs.

a. Locked wheels on bed.
b. Low beds (note that most institutional beds are 4″ to 6″ too high).
c. Increased chair height (about 22″) to ease rising from a chair. Firm pillows may be placed on seat or extenders placed on chair legs (Weiner, Long, Hughes, et al., 1993).
d. Wedge cushion placed on chair seat. Should be 4″ high at front, tapering to 1″ in midsection and 2″ in back (Johnson, 1991).
e. Ribbon or yarn draped across waist when person seated in chair as a gentle reminder to remain seated.

VI. General Staff-Based Interventions

a. Education of staff is an important component of a falls prevention program.
b. Use of Behavior Log to reveal patterns or trends (see Appendix E).
c. Placement of colored dots/stickers on the kardex, bed and intercom to identify those at highest risk for falls.
d. Close observation of new admissions and transfers for the first week.
e. Optimize staffing patterns (Cutillo-Schmitter, Rovner, & Shmuely, 1996).

(1) Novice staff need to be integrated with experienced staff. Fall rates increase when novice nurses work without expert nurses.
(2) Higher staff-to-patient ratios should be considered during the morning and evening activities of daily living.

VII. Prevention of Fall-Related Injuries

As health care providers, we also need to prevent fall-related injuries. Many of the interventions utilized for fall prevention are also beneficial in reducing fall-related injuries (Grisso, Capezuti, & Schwartz, 1996). These may include:

A. Environmental modifications, e.g., flexible flooring, wall-to-wall carpeting.
B. Use of estrogen therapy, and calcium and Vitamin D supplementation, and minimal use of psychotropic drugs.
C. A regular exercise program, and the wearing of hip pads.

VIII. Siderails

Siderails are environmental hazards which increase an older adult's risk of falling (Donius, 1995) and even death (Parker & Miles, 1997). When siderails are in the raised position, older adults may climb over them, thus increasing the risk of a serious fall. With lowered siderails, a person may easily get out of bed. Siderails are considered a restraint if they restrict an older adult's freedom of voluntary movement in and out of bed.

A. Siderail Assessment (see also Donius & Rader, 1994, for a Siderail Decision Tree).

1. Ask older adult if s/he wishes siderails to be up or down; document choice.
2. Observe person getting into and out of bed unassisted with siderails lowered and document person's ability.
3. Categorize safety risk:
   a. Level I: low risk; person able to get out of bed safely; or is unable to move and therefore is at low risk for injury.
   b. Level II: moderate risk; person wishes to get out of bed unassisted, but unable to do so safely. Other interventions are necessary.
   c. Level III: high risk; siderails are used because benefits outweigh burdens. Fall intervention strategies are also necessary.
4. Observe older adult getting into and out of bed unassisted with single half siderails elevated. If the siderail is used as an assistive device, and improves the individual's mobility, it is not considered a restraint. Note that split siderails in the elevated position are extremely hazardous. Avoid all use of 2 split rails on the same side of the bed.
5. Assessment of siderails should be ongoing.

B. Interventions designed to eliminate the need for siderails include:

1. Bed placement against wall.
2. Bed monitors.
3. Low bed, or mattress placed on floor.
4. Cushions or padding around bed.
5. Bedside commode.
6. Siderail use should be decreased in a gradual and systematic manner.
   a. May wish to switch from full siderail to single half siderail use.
   b. May determine that siderails could be lowered for specified periods, gradually eliminating use.

VIII. Summary

A fall prevention program must incorporate the philosophy of individualized care. Assessment of fall risk and implementation of appropriate interventions should be completed for each older person. Key points to remember about falls and a falls prevention program are:

A. Falls are common among older adults; however, most falls do not result in serious injury.
B. Common causes of falls include age-related changes, acute and chronic illnesses, and environmental factors.
C. Fall risk assessment includes a physical exam, medication review, laboratory evaluation, and history of previous fall(s).
D. The goal is to minimize the risk of falling or sustaining an injury, and at the same time, to maintain mobility and independence.
E. Elimination of as many fall risk factors as possible is the most promising strategy.
F. Exercise as a component of a falls prevention program is important.
G. Ongoing assessment of siderail use and elimination should be included in a fall prevention program.

A case example for Fall-Risk Assessment and a Behavior Log are included in Appendix D and E.

Bibliography

Berryman, E., Gaskin, D., Jones, A., Tolley, F., & MacMullen, J. (1989). Point by point: Predicting elders' falls. *Geriatric Nursing, 10*, 199–201.

Capezuti, E., Evans, L., Strumpf, N., & Maislin, G. (1996). Physical restraint use and falls in nursing home residents. *Journal of the American Geriatrics Society, 44*, 627–633.

Capezuti, E., Strumpf, N. E., Evans, L. K., Grisso, J. A., & Maislin, G. (1998). The relationship between physical restraint removal and falls and injuries among nursing home residents. *Journal of Gerontology: Medical Sciences, 53A*, M47–M52.

Capezuti, E., Talerico, K., Strumpf, N., & Evans, L. (1998). Individualized assessment and evaluation of bilateral siderail use. *Geriatric Nursing, 19*(6), in press.

Catchen, H. (1983). Repeater: Inpatient accidents among the hospitalized elderly. *The Gerontologist, 23*, 273–276.

Clutchins, C. (1991). Blueprint for restraint-free care. *American Journal of Nursing, 91*(7), 36–42.

Creighton, H. (1982). Law for the nurse manager: Are side rails necessary? *Nursing Management, 13*(6), 45–48.

Cutillo-Schmitter, T. A., Rovner, B. W., & Shmuely, V. (1996). Falls prevention study: A practical approach. *Journal of Healthcare Risk Management, 16*, 56–68.

DeVito, C., Lambert, D., Sattin, R., Bacchelli, S., Ros, A., & Rodriquez, J. (1988). Fall injuries among the elderly: Community-based surveillance. *Journal of the American Geriatrics Society, 36*, 1029–1035.

Donius, M. (1995). Fall prevention and management. In J. Rader & E. M. Tornquist (Eds.), *Individualized dementia care: Creative, compassionate approaches* (pp. 145–167). New York: Springer Publishing Co.

Donius, M., & Rader, J. (1994). Use of siderails: Rethinking a standard of practice. *Journal of Gerontological Nursing, 20*(11), 23–27.

Ejaz, F. K., Jones, J. A., & Rose, M. S. (1994). Falls among nursing home residents: An examination of incident reports before and after restraint reduction programs. *Journal of the American Geriatrics Society, 42*, 960–964.

Friedman, S. M., Williamson, J. D., Lee, B. H., Ankrom, M. A., Ryan, S. D., & Denman, S. J. (1995). Increased fall rates in nursing home residents after relocation to a new facility. *Journal of the American Geriatrics Society, 43*, 1237–1242.

Ginter, S. F., & Mion, L. C. (1992). Falls in the nursing home: Preventable or inevitable? *Journal of Gerontological Nursing, 18*(11), 43–48.

Glickstein, J. (Ed.), & Spector, M. [Issue Ed.] (1991). Gait and gait training in the elderly. *Focus on Geriatric Care & Rehabilitation, 4*(10), 1–8.

Granek, E., Baker, S., Abbey, H., Robinson, E., Myers, A., Samkoff, J., & Klein, L. (1987). Medications and diagnoses in relation to falls in a long-term care facility. *Journal of the American Geriatrics Society, 35*, 503–511.

Grisso, J. A., Capezuti, E., & Schwartz, A. (1996). Falls as risk factors for fractures. In R. Marcus, D. Feldman, & J. Kelsey (Eds.), *Osteoporosis* (pp. 599–611). New York: Academic Press.

Gurwitz, J. H., Sanchez-Cross, M. T., Eckler, M. A., & Matulis, J. (1994). The epidemiology of adverse and unexpected events in the long-term care setting. *Journal of the American Geriatrics Society, 42*, 33–38.

Hogue, C. C. (1992). Managing falls: The current basis for practice. In S. G. Funk, E. M. Tornquist, M. T. Champagne, & R. A. Wiese (Eds.), *Key aspects of elder care* (pp. 41–57). New York: Springer Publishing Co.

Jackson, J., & Ramsdell, J. (1989). *New Perspectives in Geriatric Medicine: Gait Disorder.* San Diego, CA: University of California, San Diego Geriatric Education Center.

Janken, J., Reynolds, B., & Swiech, K. (1986). Patient falls in the acute care setting: Identifying risk factors. *Nursing Research, 35*, 215–219.

Johnson, D. (1991). Make your own chairbound alternatives. *Geriatric Nursing, 12*, 18–20.

Lauritzen, J. B., Petersen, M. M., & Lund, B. (1993). Effect of external hip protectors on hip fractures. *The Lancet, 341*, 11–13.

Lipsitz, L., Jonsson, P., Kelley, M., & Koestner, J. (1991). Causes and correlates of recurrent falls in ambulatory frail elderly. *Journal of Gerontology: Medical Sciences, 46*, M113–M121.

Lord, S. R., Ward, J. A., Williams, P., & Strudwick, M. (1995). The effect of a 12-month exercise trial on balance, strength and falls in older women: A randomized controlled trial. *Journal of the American Geriatrics Society, 43*, 1198–1206.

Lund, C., & Sheafor, M. (1985). Is your patient about to fall? *Journal of Gerontological Nursing, 11*, 37–41.

Maki, B., Holliday, P., & Topper, A. (1991). Fear of falling and postural performance in the elderly. *Journal of Gerontology: Medical Sciences, 46*, M123–M131.

Mathias, S., Nayak, U. S. L., & Isaacs, B. (1986). Balance in the elderly patient: The "Get-up and Go" test. *Archives of Physical Medicine and Rehabilitation, 67*, 387.

Mion, L. C., Gregor, S., Buettner, M., Chwirchak, D., Lee, O., & Paras, W. (1989). Falls in the rehabilitation setting: Incidence and characteristics. *Rehabilitation Nursing, 14*(1), 17–22.

Morgan, V. R., Mathison, J. H., Rice, J. C., & Clemmer, D. I. (1985). Hospital falls: A persistent problem. *American Journal of Public Health, 75*, 775–777.

Morse, J., Tylko, S., & Dixon, H. (1987). Characteristics of the fall-prone patient. *The Gerontologist, 27*, 516–522.

Norman, G. M., & Gibbs, J. A. (1991). Clinical ambulation incentives for the immobile elderly. *Journal of Gerontological Nursing, 17*(8), 28–33.

Parker, K., & Miles, S. H. (1997). Deaths caused by siderails. *Journal of the American Geriatrics Society, 48*, 797–802.

Perry, B. (1982). Falls among the elderly: A review of the methods and conclusions of epidemiologic studies. *Journal of the American Geriatrics Society, 30*, 367–371.

Pluchino, F. (1988). Underlying cause of falls in *The older patient.* Boston, MA: The Department of Medical Research, Hebrew Rehabilitation Center for Aged.

Podsiadlo, D., & Richardson, S. (1991). The timed "Up & Go": A test of basic functional mobility for frail elderly persons. *Journal of the American Geriatrics Society, 39*, 142–148.

Province, M. A., Hadley, E. C., Hornbrook, M. C., Lipsitz, L. A., Miller, J. P., Mulrow, C. D., Ory, M. G., Sattin, R. W., Tinetti, M. E., & Wolf, S. L. (1995). The effects of exercise on falls in elderly patients: A preplanned meta-analysis of the FICSIT trials. *Journal of the American Medical Association, 273*, 1341–1347.

Rader, J., & Tornquist, E. M. (1995). *Individualized dementia care: Creative, compassionate approaches.* New York: Springer Publishing Company.

Ray, W. A., Taylor, J. A., Meador, K. G., Thapa, P. B., Brown, A. K., Kajihara, H. K., Davis, C., Gideon, P., & Griffin, M. R. (1997). A randomized trial of a consultation service to reduce falls in nursing homes. *Journal of the American Medical Association, 278*(7), 557–562.

Roberts, B. (1989). Effects of walking on balance among elders. *Nursing Research, 39*, 180–182.

Robinson, B. (1988). Evaluation of the patient who falls. *The older patient.* Boston, MA: The Department of Medical Research, Hebrew Rehabilitation Center for Aged.

Ross, J. (1991). Contributors to falls. *Journal of Gerontological Nursing, 17*(9), 19–23.

Rubenstein, L., Robbins, A., Schulmna, B., Rosado, J., Osterweil, D., & Josephson, K. (1988). Falls and instability in the elderly. *Journal of the American Geriatrics Society, 36*, 266–278.

Sabin, T. (1982). Biologic aspects of falls and mobility limitations in the elderly. *Journal of the American Geriatrics Society, 30*, 51–58.

Sklar, C. (1985). Liability for a fall. *The Canadian Nurse, May*, 15–16.

Spellbring, A., Gannon, M., Kleckner, T., & Conway, K. (1988). Improving safety for the hospitalized elderly. *Journal of Gerontological Nursing, 14*(2), 31–37.

Strumpf, N., Evans, L., & Schwartz, D. (1991). Physical restraint of the elderly. In C. Chenitz, J. Stone, & S. Salisbury (Eds.), *The clinical practice of gerontological nursing.* Philadelphia: Saunders.

Tamarin, F. (1988). Falls in the elderly: Risks and prevention. *Geriatric Medicine Today, 7*(6), 83–84.

Tideiksaar, R. (1989). *Falling in old age: Its prevention and treatment.* New York: Springer Publishing Co.

Tinetti, M. (1987). Factors associated with serious injury during falls by ambulatory nursing home residents. *Journal of the American Geriatrics Society, 35*, 644–648.

Tinetti, M., & Ginter, S. (1988). Identifying mobility dysfunction in elderly patients: Standard neuromuscular examination or direct assessment? *Journal of the American Medical Association, 259*, 1190–1193.

Tinetti, M., & Speechley, M. (1989). Prevention of falls among the elderly. *New England Journal of Medicine, 320*, 1055–1059.

Tinetti, M., Liu, W., & Ginter, S. (1992). Mechanical restraint use and fall-related injuries among residents of skilled nursing facilities. *Annals of Internal Medicine, 116*, 369–374.

Tinetti, M. E., Baker, D. I., McAvay, G., Claus, E. B., Garrett, P., Gottschalk, M., Koch, M. L., Trainor, K., & Horwitz, R. I. (1994). A multifactorial intervention to reduce the risk of falling among elderly people living in the community. *New England Journal of Medicine, 331*, 821–827.

Tinetti, M. E., Doucette, J. T., & Claus, E. B. (1995). The contributions of predisposing and situational risk factors to serious fall injuries. *Journal of the American Geriatrics Society, 43*, 1207–1213.

Tinetti, M. E., Doucette, J., Claus, E., & Marottoli, R. (1995). Risk factors for serious injury during falls by older persons in the community. *Journal of the American Geriatrics Society, 43*, 1214–1221.

van Dijk, P. T. M., Meulenberg, O. G. R. M., van de Sande, H. J., & Habbema, J. D. F. (1993). Falls in dementia patients. *The Gerontologist, 33*, 200–204.

Walshe, A., & Rosen, H. (1979). A study of patient falls from bed. *Journal of Nursing Administration, 9*(5), 31–35.

Weiner, D. K., Long, R., Hughes, M. A., Chandler, J., & Studenski, S. (1993). When older adults face the chair-rise challenge. *Journal of the American Geriatrics Society, 41*, 6–10.

Whedon, M., & Shedd, P. (1989). Prediction and prevention of patient falls. *Image: Journal of Nursing Scholarship, 21*, 108–114.

Appendix A

Risk Factors for Falls in the Elderly

I. INTRINSIC FACTORS

A. *Acute and chronic illnesses*: e.g., metabolic abnormalities, arrhythmias, orthostatic hypotension and sensory deficits.
B. *Dementia.*
C. *Incontinence.*
D. *Medications*, e.g., benzodiazepines, antipsychotics, antihistamines, cardiac drugs, antidepressants.
E. *Musculoskeletal problems*, e.g., changes or impairment in bone mass, muscle mass, muscle strength, joint function, mobility.
F. *Neurologic conditions*, e.g., seizures, strokes, Parkinson's disease.

II. EXTRINSIC FACTORS

A. *Situational*, e.g., relocation, poorly maintained or improperly used assistive devices.
B. *Environmental*, e.g., slippery floors, unstable furniture, inappropriate lighting, low toilet seats, and improper shoes and clothing.

Appendix B
Fall-Risk Assessment

- *History*: Review previous fall situation(s) for intrinsic and extrinsic factors, along with associated activities related to fall risk.
- *Medication Review*: Note recent changes in medications and use of medications associated with fall risk.
- *Physical Exam*

  — Postural vital signs
  — Mental status
  — Sensory status (vision, hearing)
  — Neurological status (muscle tone, tremors, motor strength, proprioception)
  — Musculoskeletal status (range of motion, joint deformities, feet)
  — Mobility ("Get-up and Go" or "Go Go" tests)

- *Focused Laboratory Evaluation* (e.g., CBC, electrolytes, ECG, drug levels, CT or MRI of head).

Appendix C

Profile of the Fall-Prone Older Person

1. *ADVANCED AGE*

   - Age 70 and above are at risk
   - Age 85 and older are at greatest risk

2. *ALTERED MENTAL STATUS*

   - Delirium/dementia
   - Highest risk exists with intermittent confusion

3. *ALTERED PSYCHOSOCIAL OR EMOTIONAL STATUS*

   - Agitation
   - Aggressiveness
   - Depression
   - Denial of impairment

4. *ACTUAL OR POTENTIAL INCONTINENCE*

   - Highest risk exists if independent in using toilet *and* incontinent

5. *RELOCATION*

   - New admission
   - Relocation within facility, e.g., change of room, unit, floor

6. *HISTORY OF FALLS*

   - Risk exists if 1 or 2 falls have occurred within last 6 months
   - Highest risk exists with history of multiple falls

7. *DEBILITATION OR WEAKNESS*
8. *CONFINEMENT TO CHAIR*
9. *VISUAL IMPAIRMENT(S)*
10. *POSTURAL HYPOTENSION*

    - Drop in systolic blood pressure of 20 mmHg or more between lying and standing positions

11. *ALTERED BALANCE OR GAIT*
12. *MEDICATIONS*

Anesthetics	Antidepressants	Antihistamines	Antipsychotics
Anticonvulsants	Benzodiazepines	Cardiac drugs	Cathartics
Hypoglycemics	Narcotics		

Appendix D

Case Example for Fall-Risk Assessment

Client: Rebecca Simpson

Age: 89

Problem: Frequent Falls

1. Health Status

   History

   - Mild to moderate cognitive impairment
   - Osteoarthritis
   - Bilateral cataract surgery 15 years ago

   Recent Health Problem

   - Elevated blood pressure; currently taking hydrochlorothiazide at 10:00 a.m.

   Physical Assessment

   - Pain and stiffness in hips, knees and fingers, especially in the morning
   - Posture stooped
   - Impaired range of motion in knees and hips
   - Difficulty seeing without glasses, especially in the evening and at night
   - Mild hearing loss (does not wear hearing aid)
   - Foot abnormalities (bunions, callus, a few corns, toenails thick and long)
   - Weak quadricep muscles bilaterally

2. Mental Status

- Impaired short-term memory
- Limited attention span
- Confusion worse during the evening and at night

3. Functional Status

- Needs assistance getting out of bed in morning due to pain, discomfort, and leg weakness
- Uses walker for ambulation; requires observation
- Needs assistance to bathroom for morning care; washes self seated at the sink
- Requires assistance when using the bathtub or shower
- Needs some assistance with dressing
- Once up and about, can go to the bathroom independently
- Feeds self

4. Social Status

- Widow for 20 years
- No children
- Niece visits once per week
- Retired school teacher (taught second grade for 46 years)
- Enjoys socializing; especially enjoys the company of Mr. Scott, whose room is near hers

5. Environment

Resident's room

- Lighting dim at night
- Floor uncarpeted
- Bed frequently found elevated at night

Bathroom

- Toilet of standard size and height
- Grab bars available
- Sink adjacent to toilet

Lounge/Activity room

- Chairs of varying height and design available
- Bright sunlight during the daytime, often producing glare
- Noise level varies

Hallway

- Floor surfaces uncarpeted, clean, and polished
- Handrails present

[Case can be used for discussion of risk factors and development of individualized care plan, or in conjunction with the Behavior Log, Appendix E.]

Appendix E

Behavior Log

Specific Behavior: Frequent falling from bed and chair

Client's Name: Rebecca Simpson Room # 123

Date	Exact time	What happened?	Where?	Who else was present?	What could be happening internally (*inside* client) to precipitate behavior?	What could be happening externally (*outside* client) to precipitate behavior?	What interventions help (could help) client?
1/20/97	1:00 AM	Found on floor beside bed.	Bedroom.	No one else present.	• Attempting to get to bathroom to void. • "Feet slipped." • "Bed slid away." • Poor vision • Did not call for help.	• Siderails up (full length) • Bed in high position	• Bed lowered • Bed wheels locked • Nonskid strips on floor at bedside • Night light • Call bell within reach • Bed alarm (if necessary) • 7A 1/20/97 Resident states "Nonskid strips help."

(continued)

Appendix E *(continued)*

Date	Exact time	What happened?	Where?	Who else was present?	What could be happening internally (*inside* client) to precipitate behavior?	What could be happening externally (*outside* client) to precipitate behavior?	What interventions help (could help) client?
1/25/97	11:30 AM	Fell getting up from large green lounge chair.	Activity room.	Residents: PA & RS - both watching TV. Nursing Assistant TC - talking to RS.	• Difficult to rise from chair: "Lost balance and felt weak."	• Green lounge chair too low.	• Physical therapy for strengthening exercises. • Encouraged to use smaller red lounge chair, which is better height for rising. • Walking program with incentives and awards. • 2/1/97: Observed resident rising out of red chair without difficulty.

Strumpf, N. E., & Evans, L. K. (1994–1998). *Maintaining restraint reduction in nursing homes* (1 RO1 AGO 8324). National Institute on Aging, Bethesda, MD.

6

Caring for the Person Who Interferes with Treatment

Roseanne Hanlon Rafter and Neville E. Strumpf

The Purpose of this Chapter is to:

1. Describe guidelines for care in circumstances of treatment interference.
2. Identify individualized care approaches that mimimize invasive treatments, such as feeding tubes and catheters.

I. Treatment Interference

A. Even with use of physical restraint, removal of treatment devices often occurs. Removal may be precipitated by alterations in mental status or simple discomfort with the device. Although physical restraints do not prevent treatment interference, they nevertheless are routinely applied with many treatments, including:

1. Feeding tubes (nasogastric and gastrostomy/PEG).
2. Intravenous lines.
3. Foley catheters.
4. Oxygen therapy.

5. Wound dressings.
6. Ventilators.
7. Monitoring devices.

B. When dealing with treatment interference, ethical questions should be considered. Adults must be asked their wishes regarding health care and treatment options, and such discussions need to be facilitated (Perrin, 1997). Where decision making is questioned, it is helpful for the interdisciplinary team to gather data concerning decisional capacity. Once data are collected, assessment of decisional capacity should decrease two types of errors, namely, mistakenly preventing persons who ought to be considered capacitated from directing the course of their treatment, and failing to protect incapacitated persons from the harmful effects of decisions by others (Mezey et al., 1997). Ultimately, the recommendation and selection of treatment includes weighing its potential gains versus any possible harms. Analysis of risks and benefits must take into consideration individual choice and well-being, as well as protection from harm (Reigle, 1996).

1. Potential benefits of various treatments:

   a. Treatment of health problem.
   b. Prevention of complications.
   c. Stabilization of health status.
   d. Prolongation of life when desired and desirable.
   e. Prevention of malnutrition or dehydration.
   f. Promotion of comfort.

2. Potential burdens of various treatments:

   a. Discomfort.
   b. Impersonal care associated with attention to technical devices.
   c. Reduced sense of dignity.
   d. Unnecessary prolongation of suffering and dying.
   e. Possible serious or severe complications.

C. It is important to consider therapeutic and individualized approaches that reduce the need for unnecessary or unwanted treatment. Personal wishes with regard to treatment should be ascertained and implemented to the extent possible. If invasive treatment is deemed necessary, at least on a short-term basis, approaches that decrease interference with needed treatment and promote comfort should be initiated.

II. General Guidelines for Individualized Care of Persons Receiving Various Treatments, Including Invasive Treatment (See Appendix A)

A. Select the Least Intrusive Treatment

1. Choice of treatment modality should be a collaborative decision that includes the team, older adult, and family members.
2. Consent for an invasive treatment must be obtained (preferably from the older adult) and should be clearly documented in the record.
3. The benefits and burdens of the treatment must be clear to the older adult, family, and those who review the record.

B. Explain the Treatment and Techniques to be Used

1. Interviews with older adults reveal lack of knowledge regarding treatment and purpose:

    a. "No one explained why I had this tube or how long it would be necessary."
    b. "If only someone explained what was going to happen to me."

2. Explanations may need to be repeated frequently.

C. Provide Time for Guided Exploration

1. Exploration (including with the aid of mirrors where appropriate) should be carefully guided by staff, e.g., hand-to-hand contact with tubes, dressings, etc., and supplemented with appropriate information about the treatment.
2. Familiarization with treatment devices may need frequent reinforcement to be effective.

D. Note Individual's Comfort Level

1. Discomfort may be the primary reason for treatment interference, especially when delirium, dementia, or brain lesions prevent understanding of the rationale for treatment.
2. For a person with an altered level of consciousness, treatment interference may be a purely reflexive action to a foreign (and perhaps uncomfortable) treatment device.

E. Reassess Frequently and Eliminate Invasive Treatment as Soon as Possible

1. Ongoing evaluation of the person's need for and response to the treatment is a *must*!
2. Possible reasons for discontinuing a treatment:

a. Improvement or resolution of the problem.
b. Benefits of the treatment no longer outweigh burdens:

(1) Despite treatment, the individual's condition cannot improve, e.g., irreversible terminal condition. Note that treatment interference *may* be a non-verbal sign that an individual wants the treatment stopped.
(2) The individual perceives that his or her quality of life is being impaired by continuing to receive the treatment.

3. A decision to eliminate a treatment should be clearly documented in the health care record.

F. Consider Restraint as a "Last Resort," and Adhere to the Standard in Chapter 1, Appendix B

III. Providing Individualized Care to Persons Interfering with Treatment (See Appendix B)

A. Explain Reason for the Prescribed Treatment. If possible, discuss how long the treatment may be necessary and answer any questions. Reinforce this explanation as often as necessary. Gain agreement for a short-term trial of the treatment with provisions to reassess or discontinue.
B. Guide the Person's Hand as S/he Gently Explores Any Tubing, Dressings, etc. Repeat guided exploration as frequently as necessary.

1. Tubes: Where are they going to and coming from? Lead hand from insertion or dressing site to drainage bag or other device.
2. IVs/continuous tube feedings: Point out bottle or bag hanging above or beside bed and explain or demonstrate any pump devices and alarms, if being used. Use a mirror, if helpful.
3. Endotracheal/tracheostomy tubes: How are they held in place? Guide hand around tube holder or trach ties. Show sample of trach dressing. Explain the role of the inflated cuff resting in the windpipe (trachea). What are the tubes connected to? Point out the tubing connected to the ET tube or trach; follow tubing to ventilator or oxygen source. Demonstrate ventilator alarms and sound of bellows.

C. Assure Physical Comfort with the Least Irritating Tube Placements

1. Feeding tubes (nasogastric or gastrostomy).

a. Ascertain proper tube placement.

b. Perform daily inspection and care of tube site; treat any skin irritation or infection.
c. Provide mouth and nose care each shift and PRN.
d. Assess and treat any diarrhea associated with tube feeding.

    (1) Maintain cleanliness.
    (2) Consult with dietician and physician regarding type of prescribed feeding and amounts.

e. Whenever possible, continue oral intake; periodically reassess for continued need for treatment.
f. Use commercial tube holder to stabilize and secure N-G tube.

2. Intravenous lines.

    a. Check IV site for signs of infiltration, irritation or phlebitis and infection (swelling, redness, local warmth or coldness, drainage, change in vital signs).
    b. Care for IV site daily or according to policy.
    c. Reposition extremity every 2 hours or as necessary.
    d. Provide range of motion exercises every 1-2 hours.
    e. Whenever possible, continue oral intake; periodically reassess continued need for treatment.

3. Foley catheters and drainage tubes.

    a. Ascertain tube placement, patency, and if applicable, sterility or maintenance of closed system.
    b. Perform inspection and care at insertion site daily or as prescribed; report and treat any areas of irritation or infection (redness, swelling, heat, pain, drainage, odor).
    c. Observe character of any drainage in the collection bag and report findings (amount, color, consistency, cloudiness, pus, blood, abnormal odor); infection may cause extreme discomfort and may increase the likelihood of treatment interference.

4. Oxygen equipment.

    a. Ascertain cannula or catheter placement and patency.
    b. Perform inspection and care of nose and mouth each shift and PRN.
    c. Oxygen has a drying effect on mucous membranes which become easily irritated:

        (1) A water-soluble jelly may be lightly applied to rim of the nostrils.

(2) If permissible, the person may find ice chips or hard candy helpful in relieving dry mouth.

d. Place person in a semi-Fowler's position to promote optimal lung expansion.
e. If permissible, encourage intake of water or other non-mucous producing fluids to liquefy thick lung secretions and ease coughing.

5. Dressings.

a. Change soiled dressings as frequently as necessary.
b. Note and report any signs of irritation or infection.

6. Endotracheal tubes.

a. Stabilize the endotracheal tube with a commercial tube holder (instead of traditional adhesive tape) to improve comfort and minimize the chance of self-extubation.
b. Provide adequate pain control.
c. Provide nasal and oral care every shift and as necessary.
d. Ensure that length of ventilator tubing is adequate to prevent pulling on endotracheal tube, causing discomfort for the client.
e. Adjust ventilator arms at an appropriate height to prevent tugging at endotracheal tube.
f. Ensure adequate endotracheal suctioning to maintain airway clearance and decrease discomfort related to coughing/mucus plugs.

Self-extubation by ventilator-dependent clients remains an area of concern for clinicians in acute care settings. Nevertheless, the literature presents evidence that episodes of deliberate self-extubation are actually low in number (2% to 13% of clients requiring ventilation). The rate of complications after self-extubation is also low, with associated mortality less than 1%. The percentage of clients *in physical restraints* at the time of self-extubation ranges from 41% to 91% (see numerous citations in Bibliography).

7. Tracheostomy tubes.

a. Maintain secure but comfortable trach ties.
b. Prevent irritation of skin from trach ties.
c. Change trach dressings and provide trach care frequently enough to prevent skin irritation around stoma and build-up of any mucus drainage.

d. If connected to ventilator or T-piece, ensure adequate length and flexibility of tubing for client comfort.
e. If connected to ventilator, adjust ventilator arms at appropriate height to prevent tugging at the tracheostomy.
f. Provide adequate suctioning to maintain airway clearance and prevent build-up of secretions.
g. Provide oral care as needed.
h. Provide adequate pain control.

D. Assure Psychosocial Comfort

Assuring psychosocial comfort is important in all areas of actual or potential treatment interference. For those clients requiring ventilatory support, such comfort is crucial if physical restraints are to be avoided.

With regard to self-extubation, the literature indicates that among subjects studied, agitation or restlessness was present in half of those who extubated themselves. Responding to clients who are receiving ventilatory support and dealing with their anxiety and fear is a key strategy for preventing interruption of therapy.

In addition to the anxiety associated with frightening equipment and a strange, disruptive environment, those requiring ventilatory support grapple with the devastating fear of being unable to breathe or to control their own breathing pattern. Care providers need to acknowledge the intensity of this fear and its impact on the client's ability to cope with various interventions. If clients perceive equipment and interventions as interfering with breathing, they struggle to protect themselves from such intrusions. Assisting the newly intubated client to work with, and not against, the endotracheal tube and ventilator, takes time and patience. Learning to tolerate a foreign object in one's mouth, throat, or nose requires much education and a virtual leap of faith. Acceptance of a machine to push air in and out of one's lungs is difficult physically and emotionally. Decreasing anxiety during this process requires the continual support, education, and patience of care providers.

1. Endotracheal (ETT) and tracheostomy tubes.

   a. Explain all equipment to the client and family (ETT, AmbuBag, ventilator, suction equipment, etc.).
   b. Explain all procedures (suctioning, chest physical therapy, etc.).
   c. Provide guided exploration when possible.
   d. Provide sedation judiciously.

e. Provide aids for effective communication with the client (hearing aids, eyeglasses, communication boards, writing tablets).
f. Make stressful treatments as tolerable for the client as possible.
g. Have call bell close at hand to help client feel secure in obtaining assistance or attention if needed.
h. Decrease environmental stimuli (noise, lighting, etc.) to the extent possible.
i. In a shared room, draw curtains around traumatic bedside scenes, limiting exposure to upsetting, anxiety-producing events.
j. Remove malodorous objects and substances from the environment as soon as possible.
k. Provide reality cues such as calendars, watches, or clocks.
l. Encourage family and friends to remain at the bedside (as it is reasonable) to decrease loneliness and isolation. (Availability of others at the bedside can help prevent interruption of therapy without resorting to physical restraint.)
m. Include the client's family/significant others in care planning.
n. Provide soothing, quiet music. Use headset if needed.
o. Provide diversional activities such as audiotapes of books, radio and TV programs, or reading by visitors.
p. Facilitate visits from clergy if client desires. Fears concerning death and dying may be explored and other spiritual needs met.
q. Maintain a calm, quiet, soothing tone of voice. Use gentle touch and movements when working with the client.
r. Make the environment more familiar and comforting by encouraging family pictures, small personal mementoes, or religious objects as desired.
s. Include the client in care planning and encourage as much input as possible.
t. Be attuned to times when weaning may be successfully initiated.

E. Camouflage and Proper Maintenance of Treatment Site

1. Feeding tubes (gastrostomy/PEG tubes):

   Consider an abdominal binder (not too tight) or form-fitting undergarments, long pull-on tee or spandex shirts, etc.

2. Intravenous lines:

   a. Consider protective sleeves, a wrist band, e.g., type worn by athletes, loose gauze, stockinette; remove and inspect beneath camouflage regularly to detect problems.

b. Short-term use of an air splint to prevent bending at the elbow, or gloves, mitts, or socks over the person's hand; digit extenders may be appropriate.

3. Foley catheters/drainage tubes can be camouflaged with:

   a. Undergarments.
   b. Loose binders (not appropriate for Foley catheters).
   c. Slip-on shirts or sweaters.

4. Dressings:

   Consider camouflaging with outer clothing whenever possible.

F. Provide Appropriate Diversional Activity

The type of diversional activity available will be influenced by the clinical setting, acuity of the client, and availability of recreational and activity staff. Family members and friends may assist with diversional activity, in addition to staff, aides, and volunteers. Examples of diversionary activities include:

1. Music (consider a head set).
2. Books, magazines and audiotapes.
3. Something to hold, such as a religious object, a hug pillow, foam ball, or stuffed animal.
4. Conversation.
5. Scheduled conversation or reading provided by family, friends, or volunteers.

G. Encourage Involvement in Appropriate Activity Programs

In those facilities where a formalized activity program is in place, and recreational or activity staff available, additional options for diversional activities are possible:

1. Group discussions.
2. Reminiscence groups.
3. Sing-a-longs.

Note that certain treatments place restrictions on participating in activity programs, e.g., IV lines may preclude joining in exercise groups. When activities are varied, however, people can and should be helped and encouraged to attend those suitable to the situation. Recreational and activity staff should be contributing to the care plan for actual or potential treatment interference.

H. Teach and Involve Older Adult and Family in the Plan of Care
I. Reassess the Person's Need for Continued Treatment on a Regular Basis and Discontinue Treatment as Soon as Possible
J. Assess for and Promptly Treat any Reversible Changes in Mental Status Which May Influence Acceptance or Rejection of Treatment

1. Acute exacerbation of a chronic condition.
2. Medications.
3. Acute illness, infection, etc.

K. When Interventions are Unsuccessful, Choose the Least Restrictive Option to Limit Treatment Interference and Discontinue as Soon as Possible

1. Garden gloves.
2. Ski mitts.
3. Other hand mitts.
4. Air splints.
5. Digit extenders.

IV. When dealing with actual or potential treatment interference, interventions other than physical restraint can be utilized. Preventive approaches include:

A. Early Detection of Problems

1. Method: Ongoing individualized assessment.
2. Key observations:

   a. Are basic physical needs adequately met, e.g., need for food, water, activity, rest, etc.?
   b. Have there been recent changes in physical condition?
   c. Are psychological, social, and emotional needs being met?
   d. Are there recent changes in behavior?

B. Early Diagnosis

1. Method: Investigate and make sense of behavioral changes (remember that all behavior is meaningful); Behavior Log may be helpful.
2. Key domains for assessment:

   a. Physical health and functional status.
   b. Psychosocial or mental/emotional status.

c. Environmental conditions.

C. Individualized Care for Specific Problems (as described in D, E, F, and G below)

D. Individualized Approaches in Cases of Limited Fluid Intake (See Appendix C)

1. Early detection—Observe for:

a. Decreased skin turgor.
b. Dry mucous membranes.
c. Decreased urine output.
d. Changes in mental status.
e. Change in baseline vital signs.
f. Change in character of bowel movement, e.g., loose, hard.
g. Abnormalities in lab values.

2. Other considerations:

a. Fluids hard to reach or obtain?
b. Fluid dislikes?
c. Difficulty speaking or expressing thirst?
d. Heavy consumption of drinks with caffeine?
e. Medication side effects or other interactions?
f. Medical problems?

3. Early intervention—Examples:

a. Assure 24-hour intake of at least 1,500 ml (unless contraindicated).
b. Don't wait for complaints of thirst, which are likely to be a late symptom of dehydration in older adults.
c. Offer a variety of fluids based on preferences, ability to swallow, any dietary restrictions and at desired temperatures, e.g., water, fruit juice, jello, custards/puddings, ice pops.
d. Monitor or limit coffee and other drinks containing caffeine. Caffeine acts as a diuretic and may require additional fluid intake.
e. Offer fluids frequently (hourly), including fluids with afternoon and evening snacks.
f. Offer larger containers of fluids with meals and medications.
g. Provide cups, glasses, and pitchers that are easy to handle; assist as needed.
h. Provide mouth care after eating.
i. Review medications; be alert to drugs which may cause fluid loss.

j. Replace fluid if the person has been febrile, diaphoretic, has had diarrhea, etc.
k. Teach the person and family members specific amounts and types of fluids to take daily.

E. Individualized Approaches in Cases of Limited Nutritional Intake (See Appendix D)

1. Early detection—Observe for:

a. Consistent refusal to eat 50% or more of 2 meals per day.
b. Recent weight loss.
c. Weight less than 80% of desirable body weight.
d. Biochemical changes:

(1) Hemoglobin < 12 g/dl for men and < 10 g/dl for women.
(2) Serum albumin < 200 mg/dl.
(3) Total lymphocyte count < 800.
(4) Serum transferrin < 30 g/dl.

2. Other considerations:

a. Loss or poor condition of teeth?
b. Poor mouth care?
c. Inactivity?
d. Immobility?
e. Psychosocial or emotional status:

(1) New admission?
(2) Limited socialization or companionship?
(3) Depression?
(4) Incontinence (accompanied by low self-esteem and embarrassment)?

f. Medication side effects or other interactions?
g. Requires more time to finish meals or needs assistance?
h. Medical problems?
i. Difficulty swallowing?

3. Early intervention—Examples:

a. Consult with dentist.
b. Provide mouth care before each meal as necessary.
c. Allow opportunity for elimination 15–30 minutes before meals.

Esdort to dining room for each meal to encourage social interaction.

e. Establish agreeable seating pattern in dining room.
f. Offer food early or first to provide a longer meal time if the person eats slowly.
g. Assist with feeding as necessary, allowing sufficient time for chewing of food.
h. Encourage participation in at least one activity program per day.
i. Encourage intake by gentle verbal reminders to eat, given with light touch on the forearm.

F. Individualized Approaches in Cases of Difficulty Swallowing (Donahue, 1990) (See Appendix E)

1. Early detection—Observe for:

   a. Vertical movement of neck muscles as the person forces a swallow.
   b. Packing of food in cheeks.
   c. Drooling.
   d. Coughing or effort to clear throat, especially after a swallow.
   e. Absent or weak cough.
   f. Fluid leaking from nose after a swallow.
   g. Absent or weak gag reflex.

2. Other considerations:

   a. Improper positioning.
   b. Medical problems:

      (1) CVA.
      (2) Head trauma.
      (3) Cancer (throat, esophagus, lung, etc.).
      (4) Nerve or muscle disease.

3. Early intervention—Examples:

   a. Consult with specialist as necessary, e.g., physiatrist, speech therapist.
   b. Provide supervised eating especially for new clients (at least 3 meals) to identify swallowing difficulty.
   c. Be prepared for choking:

      (1) Management of the choking victim (Heimlich maneuver).

(2) Suction machine.
(3) Portable oxygen.

d. Position properly:

(1) Sit erect.
(2) Lean slightly forward.
(3) Head flexed forward.

e. Place food onto unaffected side of tongue (if applicable); press down gently on tongue and rock spoon back and forth (helps deposit food on tongue).

f. Provide step-by-step guidance and demonstration:

(1) Open mouth.
(2) Allow food to be felt on tongue.
(3) Taste the food.
(4) Chew.
(5) Lift tongue to the roof of mouth.
(6) Hold lips closed (this may have to be done *for* the person or taught).
(7) Put chin down.
(8) Swallow (it may be helpful to massage the throat slightly on the affected side to help stimulate the swallow reflex).
(9) Swallow again (this encourages more complete clearance of the throat).
(10) Relax.

g. Take time; don't ask the person to speak until a few seconds after swallowing (as speaking risks aspiration):

(1) Sit down.
(2) Convey that there is enough time.

h. Use finger (person's or your own) to clear food out of cheek if food packing is a problem.

i. Administer liquids cautiously, especially clear or thin liquids (they may be more difficult to swallow).

j. Maintain sitting position for at least 15 minutes after eating.

G. Individualized Approaches in Cases of Urinary Incontinence (See Appendix F)

1. Early detection—Observe for:

a. Inability to hold urine long enough to get to bathroom or use bedside equipment.
b. Bed, chair, floor, or clothing soiled with urine.

2. Other considerations:

a. Urinary tract infection?
b. Fecal impaction?
c. Great distance to bathroom or commode?
d. Mobility problems?
e. Inability to manipulate clothing?
f. Inadequate fluids?
g. Altered mental status?
h. Medication side effects or other interactions?
i. Medical problems:

(1) Obstruction.
(2) Nervous system disorder.
(3) Muscular problem.

3. Early intervention—Examples:

a. Treat underlying and reversible health problems.
b. Establish schedule for use of toilet, commode, bedpan, or urinal.
c. Re-evaluate and adjust medication or time of administration if possible.
d. Label bathroom doors.
e. Decrease distance to bathroom.
f. Ask family about clothing adaptations.
g. Consult with physical therapy regarding muscle strengthening exercises.
h. Encourage fluids.
i. Obtain continence evaluation or consultation for pelvic floor exercise.

V. Case Study with Behavior Logs (See Appendix G–K)
VI. Summary

Caring for persons who interfere with treatment is a challenge in any clinical setting. Weighing the benefits of treatment against associated risks needs to occur early in the clinical decision-making process. Utilizing individualized approaches can promote restraint-free care. When potentially distressing treatments appear necessary, incorporation of clinical guidelines and approaches to care may eliminate the use of restraints. When dealing with treatment interference, key points to remember are:

1. Interference with treatment occurs for a variety of reasons; a careful assessment of the problem is essential.
2. There are no easy answers to the difficult questions associated with maintenance of treatments and technologies; every person must be considered individually.
3. Interventions can be employed to facilitate treatment maintenance. These interventions are based on:

    a. Individualized care.
    b. Attention to physical and psychosocial comfort.
    c. Prompt treatment of underlying problems.

4. Knowledge of individual advance directives concerning treatment decisions are extremely helpful. In ascertaining individual preferences regarding treatment, the subject of physical restraint to maintain such treatment should also be discussed.

Bibliography

Adams, F. (1988). Fluid intake: How much do elders drink? *Geriatric Nursing*, *9*, 218–220.

Barclay, B. A., & Litchford, M. D. (1991). Incidence of nasoduodenal tube occlusion and patient removal of tubes: A prospective study. *Journal of the American Dietetic Association, 91*, 220–222.

Barr, W. J. (1996). Do restraints really protect intubated patients? *American Journal of Nursing, 96*(6), 51.

Bizek, K. (1995). Optimizing sedation in critically ill, mechanically ventilated patients. *Critical Care Nursing Clinics of North America*, *7*, 315–325.

Bizek, K., Freeman, L., Natale, P., & Kruse, J. (1991). Factors influencing unplanned extubations in the intensive care unit.[Abstract]. *Heart and Lung, 20*(4), 24A.

Brown, R., Grau, P., & Touleimat, B. (1992). Unplanned extubation in a community hospital.[Abstract]. *CHEST, 102*(2), 183S.

Ciocon, J. 0., Silverstone, F. A., Graver, M., & Foley, C. J. (1988). Tube feedings in elderly patients: indications, benefits, and complications. *Archives of Internal Medicine, 148,* 429–433.

Ciocon, J. 0., Galindo-Ciocon, D. J., Thiessen, C., & Galindo, D. (1992). Comparison of intermittent vs. continuous tube feeding among the elderly. *Journal of Parenteral Enteral Nutrition, 16*, 525–528.

Cooper, M. C. (1993). The intersection of technology and care in the ICU. *Advances in Nursing Science, 15*(3), 23–32.

Cooper, M. C. (1994). Care: Antidote for nurses' love-hate relationship with technology. *American Journal of Critical Care, 3*, 402–403.

Coppolo, D. P., & May, J. J. (1990). Self-extubations: A 12-month experience. *CHEST, 105,* 1804–1807.

Creditor, M. C. (1993). Hazards of hospitalization of the elderly. *Annals of Internal Medicine, 118,* 219–223.

Donahue, P. (1990). When it's hard to swallow: Feeding techniques for dysphagia management. *Journal of Gerontological Nursing, 16*(4), 6–9.

Eaton, M., Mitchell-Bonair, I. L., & Iriedman, E. (1986). The effect of touch on nutritional intake of chronic organic brain syndrome patients. *Journal of Gerontology, 4,* 611–616.

Eberts, M., & Taggart, J. (1991). Unplanned endotracheal extubation: incidence and contributing factors. (Abstract]. *Heart and Lung, 20*(4), 23A.

Editorial. (1989). Understanding the benefits and burdens of tube feedings. *Archives of Internal Medicine, 149,* 1925–1926.

Ellstrom, K., Brenner, M., & Williams, J. (1991). Incidence and factors related to unplanned extubation in the intensive care unit. [Abstract]. *Heart and Lung, 20*(4),23A.

Evans, L. K., & Strumpf, N. E. (1989). Tying down the elderly: A review of the literature on physical restraint use. *Journal of the American Geriatric Society, 37,* 65–74.

Evans, L. K., Strumpf, N. E., & Williams, C. C. (1992). Limiting the use of physical restraints: a prerequisite to independent function. In E. Calkins, A. Ford, & P. Katz (Eds.), *The practice of geriatrics* (pp. 204–210). (2nd ed.) Philadelphia: W. B. Saunders Co.

Fleming, C. (1992). The patient who refused to be fed. In G. B. White (Ed.), *Ethical dilemmas in contemporary nursing practice* (pp. 1–12). Washington, DC: American Nurses Publishing.

Fletcher, K., (1996). Use of restraints in the elderly. *AACN Clinical Issues, 7*(4), 611–620.

Fowler, M. (1990). Reflections on ethics consultation in critical care settings. *Critical Care Nursing Clinics of North America, 2*(3) 431–435.

Frengley, J. D., & Mion, L. C. (1986). Incidence of physical restraints on acute general medical wards. *Journal of the American Geriatric Society, 34,* 565–568.

Galindo-Ciocon, D. J. (1993). Tube feeding: Complications among the elderly. *Journal of Gerontological Nursing, 19*(6), 17–22.

Gaspar, P. (1988). Fluid intake: What determines how much patients drink? *Geriatric Nursing,* 221–224.

Grad, A., & Jorgensen, S. (1990). A descriptive study of the incidence and factors related to unplanned extubations in critically ill adult medical patients. [Abstract]. *Heart and Lung, 19*(3), 306.

Grap, M. J., Glass, C., & Lindamood, M. O. (1995). Factors related to unplanned extubation of endotracheal tubes. *Critical Care Nurse, 15*(2), 57–65.

Hall-Lord, M. L., Larsson, G., & Bostrom, I. (1994). Elderly patients' experiences of pain and distress in intensive care: a grounded theory study. *Intensive and Critical Care Nursing, 10,* 133–141.

Happ, M. E. (1998). A grounded theory study of treatment interference in critically ill older adults. Ann Arbor, MI: UMI Dissertation Services.

Hogstel, M., & Robinson, N. (1990). Feeding the frail elderly. *Journal of Gerontological Nursing, 15*(3), 16–20.

Holly, C. M. (1993). The ethical quandaries of acute care nursing practice. *Journal of Professional Nursing, 9*(2), 110–115.

Jablonski, R. S. (1994). The experience of being mechanicallv ventilated. *Qualitative Health Research, 4*(2), 186–207.

Jayamanne, D., Nandipati, R., & Patel, D. (1988). Self-extubation: a prospective study. *CHEST* [Suppl], *98*, 3S.

Johns, J. L. (1996). Advance directives and opportunities for nurses. *IMAGE: Journal of Nursing Scholarship, 28*(2), 149–153.

Kanski, G. W., Janelli, L. M., Jones, H. M., & Kennedy, M. C. (1996). Family reactions to restraints in an acute care setting. *Journal of Gerontological Nursing, 22*(6), 17–22.

Kayser-Jones, J. (1996). Mealtime in nursing homes: The importance of individualized care. *Journal of Gerontological Nursing, 22*(3), 26–31.

Kayser-Jones, J., & Schell, E. (1997). The mealtime experience of a cognitively impaired elder: Ineffective and effective strategies. *Journal of Gerontological Nursing, 23*(7), 33–39.

Listello, D. & Sessler, C. N. (1994). Unplanned extubation: clinical predictors for reintubation. *CHEST, 105*, 1496–1503.

Macpherson, D. S., Lofgren, R. P., Granieri, R., & Myllenbeck, S. (1990). Deciding to restrain medical patients. *Journal of the American Geriatrics Society, 38*, 516–520.

Mezey, M., Mitty, E., & Ramsey, G. (1997). Assessment of decision-making capacity, nursing's role. *Journal of Gerontological Nursing, 23*(3), 28–35.

Mion, L. (1996). Establishing alternatives to physical restraint in the acute care setting: A conceptual framework to assist nurses' decision-making. *AACN Clinical Issues, 7*(4), 592 602.

Michaelsson, E., Norberg, A., & Norberg, B. (1987). Feeding methods for demented patients in end stage of life. *Geriatric Nursing, 8*, 69–73.

Norberg, A., Norberg, B., & Bexell, G. (1980). Ethical problems in feeding patients with advanced dementia. *British Medical Journal, 28l*, 847–848.

Ortiz-Pruitt, J. (1995). Physical restraint of critically ill patients. *Critical Care Nursing Clinics of North America, 7*(2), 363–373.

Ouimet-Perrin, K. (1997). Giving voice to the wishes of elders. *Journal of Gerontological Nursing, 23*(3), 18–27.

Perisi, A. J. (1994). Two-year study of the prevention of unintentional extubation. *Critical Care Nursing Quarterly, 17*(3), 35–39.

Perisi, A. J., Stuart, K., Kobe, E., & Stewart, W. (1990). Protocol for prevention of unintentional extubation. *Critical Care Nursing Quarterly, 12*(4), 87–90.

Porter, L. A. (1995). Procedural distress in critical care settings. *Critical Care Nursing Clinics of North America, 7*(2), 307–314.

Quill, T. (1989). Utilization of nasogastric feeding tubes in a group of chronically ill, elderly patients in a community hospital. *Archives of Internal Medicine, 149*, 1937–1941.

Reedy, D. (1988). Fluid intake: How can you prevent dehydration? *Geriatric Nursing*, 224–226.

Reigle, J. (1996). The ethics of physical restraints in critical care. *AACN Clinical Issues, 7*(4), 585–591.

Robbins, L. G., Boyko, E., Lane, J., Cooper, D., & Jahnigen, D. W. (1987). Binding the elderly: a prospective study of the use of mechanical restraints in an acute care hospital. *Journal of the American Geriatrics Society, 35*, 290–296.

Robinson, B. E., Sucholeiki, R., & Schocken, D. D. (1993). Sudden death and resisted mechanical restraint: A case report. *Journal of the American Geriatrics Society, 41*, 424–425.

Scherer, Y. K., Janelli, L. M., Wu, Y. B., & Kuhn, M. M. (1993). Restrained patients: An important issue for critical care nursing. *Heart & Lung, 22*, 77–83.

Seudal, I., Garner, C. V., & Kaye, W. (1992). Accidental extubation in the ICU. *CHEST, 102*, 184S.

Weaver, J. (1989). Denied more than his donuts. *American Journal of Nursing, 84*(10), 1273–1274.

Whelan, J., Simpson, S. Q., & Levy, H. (1994). Unplanned extubation; predictors of successful termination of mechanical ventilatory support. *CHEST, 105*, 1808–1812.

Wilkinson, P. (1992). The influence of high technology care on patients, their relatives and nurses, *Intensive and Critical Care Nursing, 8*, 194–198.

Wilson, E. B. (1996). Physical restraint of elderly patients in critical care. *Critical Care Nursing Clinics of North America, 8*(1) 61–70.

Appendix A

General Guidelines for Individualized Care of Persons Receiving Various Treatments, Including Invasive Treatment

- Select the least intrusive treatment possible.
- Explain the treatment and techniques to be used.
- Provide time for guided exploration.
- Note individual's comfort level.
- Reassess frequently and eliminate invasive treatment as soon as possible.
- Consider physical restraint as a "last resort."

Appendix B

Summary of Individualized Care for Persons Interfering with Treatment

1. Explain reason for the prescribed treatment.

2. Guide the person's hand as s/he gently explores any tubing, dressings, etc., and repeat exploration as frequently as necessary. Use mirror as appropriate.

3. Assure physical comfort with least irritating tube placements.

   - Feeding tubes (nasogastric/gastrostomy):

     Ascertain proper tube placement.
     Perform daily inspection and care of tube site; treat any skin irritation or infection.
     Provide mouth and nose care each shift and PRN.
     Assess and treat any diarrhea associated with tube feeding.
     Whenever possible, continue oral intake; periodically reassess continued need for treatment.
     Use commercial tube holder to stabilize and secure N-G tube.

   - Intravenous lines:

     Check IV site regularly.
     Care for IV site daily or according to policy.
     Reposition extremity every 2 hours or as necessary.
     Provide range of motion exercises every 1–2 hours.
     Whenever possible, continue oral intake; periodically reassess continued need for treatment.

- Foley catheters and drainage tubes:

  Ascertain tube placement, patency, and sterility/cleanliness.
  Perform inspection and care at insertion site daily or as prescribed.
  Observe character of any drainage and report findings.

- Oxygen equipment:

  Ascertain cannula or catheter placement and patency.
  Perform inspection and care of nose and mouth each shift and PRN.
  Counter the drying effects of oxygen on mucous membranes which become easily irritated.
  Place person in semi-Fowler's position.
  If permissible, encourage intake of water or other non-mucous producing fluids.

- Dressings:

  Change soiled dressings as frequently as necessary.
  Note and report any signs of irritation or infection.

- Endotracheal tubes:

  Stabilize endotracheal tube with a commercial tube holder.
  Provide adequate pain control.
  Provide nasal and oral care.
  Ensure that length of ventilator tubing is adequate.
  Adjust ventilator arms at an appropriate height.
  Ensure adequate endotracheal suctioning.

- Tracheostomy tubes:

  Maintain secure but comfortable trach ties.
  Prevent irritation of skin from trach ties.
  Change trach dressings and provide trach care frequently.
  If connected to ventilator or T-piece, ensure adequate length and flexibility of tubing.
  If connected to ventilator, adjust ventilator arms at appropriate height.
  Provide adequate suctioning.
  Provide oral care as needed.
  Provide adequate pain control.

4. Assure psychosocial comfort:

- Endotracheal and tracheostomy tubes:

  Explain all equipment to client and family.
  Explain all procedures.
  Provide guided exploration when possible.
  Provide sedation judiciously.
  Provide aids for effective communication.
  Make stressful treatments as tolerable as possible.
  Have call bell close at hand.
  Decrease environmental stimuli to extent possible.
  Limit visualization of traumatic bedside scenes.
  Remove malodorous objects and substances.
  Provide reality cues.
  Encourage family/significant others to remain at the bedside (as reasonable).
  Include family/significant others in care planning.
  Provide soothing, quiet music.
  Provide diversional activities to the extent possible.
  Facilitate visits from clergy as desired.
  Maintain a calm, quiet, soothing tone of voice. Use gentle touch and movements.
  Personalize the environment as possible.
  Include the client in care planning.
  Be attuned to possible weaning.

5. Camouflage and proper maintenance of treatment site.

   - Feeding tubes (gastrostomy/PEG tubes):

     Consider an abdominal binder (not too tight) or form-fitting undergarments, long pull-on tee or spandex shirts, etc.

   - Intravenous lines:

     Consider protective sleeves or wrist band.
     Use of an air splint to prevent bending at the elbow, or gloves, mitts, or socks over the hand.

   - Foley catheters/drainage tubes:

     Camouflage with:

     Undergarments
     Loose binders (not appropriate for Foley catheters)

Slip on shirts or sweaters.

- Dressings:

  Camouflage with outer clothing whenever possible.

6. Provide appropriate diversional activity and activity programs.
7. Teach and involve client/family in plan of care.
8. Reassess need for treatment and discontinue as soon as possible.
9. Assess for and promptly treat any reverisble changes in mental status.
10. When interventions are unsuccessful, choose the least restrictive option to limit treatment interference (gloves, mitts, splints, etc.) and discontinue as soon as possible.

Appendix C

Individualized Approaches in Cases of Limited Fluid Intake

Early Detection—Observe for:	Other Considerations:	Early Intervention—Examples:
• Decreased skin turgor • Dry mucous membranes • Decreased urine output • Changes in mental status • Change in baseline vital signs • Change in character of bowel movement • Abnormalities in lab values	• Fluids hard to reach or obtain • Fluid dislikes • Difficulty speaking or expressing thirst • Heavy consumption of drinks with caffeine • Medication side effects and other interactions • Medical problems	• Assure 24-hour intake of at least 1,500 ml (unless contraindicated). • Don't wait for complaints of thirst. • Offer a variety of fluids as indicated by preference and condition. • Monitor or limit coffee and other drinks containing caffeine. • Offer fluids frequently (hourly). • Offer larger containers of fluids with meals and medications. • Provide cups, glasses, and pitchers that are easy to handle, and assist as needed. • Provide mouth care after eating. • Review drugs which may cause fluid loss. • Replace fluid if febrile, diaphoretic, diarrhea, etc. • Teach the person and family members specific amounts and types of fluids to take daily.

Appendix D

Individualized Approaches in Cases of Limited Nutritional Intake

Early Detection— Observe for:	Other Considerations:	Early Intervention—Examples:
• Consistent refusal to eat 50% or more of 2 meals per day • Recent weight loss • Weight less than 80% of desirable body weight • Biochemical changes -Hemoglobin <12g/dl for men <10g/dl for women -Serum albumin <200 mg/dl -Total lymphocyte ct. <800 -Serum transferrin <30 g/dl	• Loss or poor condition of teeth • Poor mouth care • Inactivity • Immobility • Psychosocial or emotional status: -new admission -limited socialization/ companionship -depression -incontinence with low self-esteem or embarrassment • Medication side effects and other interactions • Requires more time to finish meals or needs assistance • Medical problems • Difficulty swallowing	• Consult with dentist. • Provide mouth care before each meal and as necessary. • Allow opportunity for elimination 15-30 minutes before meals. • Escort to dining room for each meal to encourage social interaction. • Establish agreeable room seating pattern in dining room. • Offer food early or first to provide a longer meal time if the person eats slowly. • Assist with feeding as necessary, allowing sufficient time for chewing of food. • Encourage participation in at least one activity program per day. • Encourage intake by gentle verbal reminders to eat, given with light touch on the forearm.

Appendix E

Individualized Approaches in Cases of Difficulty in Swallowing

Early Detection—Observe for:	Other Considerations:	Early Intervention—Examples:
• Vertical movement of neck muscles as the person forces a swallow • Packing of food in cheeks • Drooling • Cough or effort to clear throat, especially after a swallow • Absent or weak cough • Fluid leaking from nose after a swallow • Absent or weak gag reflex	• Improper positioning • Medical Problems: stroke (CVA) head trauma cancer diseases of nervous or muscular systems	• Consult with specialist as necessary, e.g., physiatrist, speech therapist. • Provide supervised eating especially for new clients (at least 3 meals) to identify swallowing difficulty. • Be prepared for choking: Management of the choking victim (Heimlich maneuver). Suction machine. Portable oxygen. • Position properly: Sit erect. Lean slightly forward. Head flexed forward. • Place food onto unaffected side of tongue (if applicable); press down gently on tongue and rock spoon back and forth (helps deposit food on tongue). • Provide step-by-step guidance and demonstration: Open mouth. Allow food to be felt on tongue. Taste food.

Early Detection—Observe for:	Other Considerations:	Early Intervention—Examples:
		Chew. Lift tongue to roof of mouth. Hold lips closed (this may have to be done for the person or taught). Put chin down. Swallow (it may be helpful to massage the throat slightly on the affected side to help stimulate the swallow reflex). Swallow again (this encourages more complete clearance of the throat). Relax. • Take time; don't ask the person to speak until a few seconds after swallowing (speaking risks aspiration): Sit down. Convey that there is enough time. • Use finger (client's or your own) to clear food out of cheek if food packing is a problem. • Administer liquids cautiously, especially clear or thin liquids; these may be more difficult to swallow. • Maintain sitting position for at least 15 minutes after eating.

Source: Donahue, P. (1990). When it's hard to swallow. *Journal of Gerontological Nursing*, *16*(4), 6–9.

Appendix F

Individualized Approaches in Cases of Urinary Incontinence

Early Detection—Observe for:	Other Considerations:	Early Intervention—Examples:
• Inability to hold urine • Bed, chair, floor or clothing soiled with urine	• Urinary tract infection • Fecal impaction • Great distance to bathroom or commode • Mobility problems • Inability to manipulate clothing • Inadequate fluids • Altered mental status • Medication side effects or other interactions • Medical problems: Obstruction Nervous system disorder Muscular problem	• Treat underlying and reversible health problems. • Establish schedule for use of toilet, commode, bedpan, or urinal. • Re-evaluate and adjust medication or time of administration if possible. • Label bathroom doors. • Decrease distance to bathroom. • Ask family about clothing adaptations. • Consult with physical therapy regarding muscle strengthening exercises. • Encourage fluids. • Obtain continence evaluation or consultation for pelvic floor exercises.

Appendix G

Case Study

Part I

Directions: Refer to Behavior Log 1 (Appendix H) for details of an episode in which Mrs. Scott's nasogastric tube was found lying on the floor. Identify approaches that might be used to decrease or eliminate (a) Mrs. Scott's attempts to dislodge the tube and (b) physical restraint.

Mrs. Scott, 84 years old, has been a nursing home resident for 1 year. She has Alzheimer's disease (early stage) and is mildly confused. Over a period of 3 months, Mrs. Scott lost considerable weight and, despite the staff's efforts to improve her nutritional intake, continued to refuse most foods and fluids.

Mrs. Scott was eventually evaluated and treated in the hospital for a duodenal ulcer. She has been readmitted to the nursing home but continues to refuse food. The staff notice that she is becoming weaker and less mobile and that her skin is beginning to show early signs of pressure ulcer formation. The staff and Mrs. Scott's family collaboratively made the decision to begin a trial of nasogastric tube feeding. On numerous occasions, the nasogastric tube has been found lying on the floor at the bedside and subsequently, wrist restraints were applied. Mrs. Scott is no longer mildly confused; instead she is distressed to the point of being hostile and aggressive with the staff and her overall confusion is noticeably worse.

Part II

Directions: Refer to Behavior Log 2 (Appendix I) for details of an episode in which Mrs. Scott was observed to be picking and pulling at the gastrostomy tube. Share ideas about responses to this new situation.

Mrs. Scott eventually has a gastrostomy tube inserted. Shortly after the tube is placed, the staff find Mrs. Scott picking at the tube site.

Part III

Directions: Refer to Behavior Log 3 (Appendix J) for details of an episode in which Mrs. Scott was found pulling at her endotracheal tube with the adhesive strips already removed from her face. Discuss possible responses to pulling at the endotracheal tube, and possible extubation.

Mrs. Scott's health status has deteriorated and she has become less mobile, resisting any attempts to transfer to a chair or ambulation. She has developed bilateral pneumonia and related hypoxia. She has been transferred to an acute care facility where she is currently intubated. Mrs. Scott is placed on a respirator for ventilatory support. The night nurse finds Mrs. Scott pulling at her endotracheal tube after removing the adhesive tapes from her face.

Part IV

Directions: Refer to Behavior Log 4 (Appendix K) for details of an episode in which Mrs. Scott pulled at the tracheostomy ties until the ties came undone, dislodging the dressing. Identify approaches that can be used to eliminate interference with the tracheostomy and dressings.

Mrs. Scott was transferred back to the nursing home with a tracheostomy tube leading to a T-piece for supplemental oxygen. A gastrostomy tube remains in place for enteral nutrition.

As an additional exercise, discuss the ethical implications of this trajectory of events.

Appendix H

Behavior Log 1: Removal of Nasogastric Tube

Specific Behavior: Removal of nasogastric tube

Client's Name: M. Scott Room # 123

Date	Exact time	What happened?	Where?	Who else was present?	What could be happening internally (*inside* client) to precipitate behavior?	What could be happening externally (*outside* client) to precipitate behavior?	What interventions help (could help) client?
1/9/98	9:30 AM	NG tube on floor at bedside. Very agitated. Pulling at wrist restraint on left hand, crying, "Unlock me."	Resident's room.	No one else present.	Agitation and confusion related to discomfort from NG tube.	Nasal secretions crusted around the tube. Application of wrist restraint on right hand. Nares sore and reddened. Mouth dry. NPO.	Explain reason for treatment. Remove wrist restraint and provide guided exploration of NG tube entry and connection to feeding pump. Demonstrate pump alarm, explaining what alarm means.

continued

Appendix H *(continued)*

Date	Exact time	What happened?	Where?	Who else was present?	What could be happening internally (*inside* client) to precipitate behavior?	What could be happening externally (*outside* client) to precipitate behavior?	What interventions help (could help) client?
							Provide nasal care q shift. Provide mouth care q2-4 hrs. Ask physician about providing supplemental oral foods and fluids.Reinforce explanation. Use a short trial of ski gloves or hand mitts if above efforts are unsuccessful. (Note needs for periodic observation, removal of mitts, etc.)

Strumpf, N. E., & Evans, L. K. (1994–1998). *Maintaining restraint reduction in nursing homes* (1 RO1 AGO 8324). Bethesda, MD: National Institute on Aging.

Appendix I

Behavior Log 2: Picking at Gastrostomy Tube Site

Specific Behavior: Picking at gastrostomy tube site

Client's Name: M. Scott   Room # 123

Date	Exact time	What happened?	Where?	Who else was present?	What could be happening internally (*inside* client) to precipitate behavior?	What could be happening externally (*outside* client) to precipitate behavior?	What interventions help (could help) client?
1/20/98	2:30 PM	Picking and pulling at gastrostomy tube.	Lounge.	Charge nurse and nursing assistant.	Lacks understanding (States: "What is this thing"?) May be experiencing discomfort at site.	Gastrostomy performed 2 days ago. Small amount serous drainage at GT site. Skin around tube may be excoriated.	Explain treatment. Guided exploration. Inspect tube site daily; cleanse and keep free from irritating drainage.

(continued)

Appendix I *(continued)*

Date	Exact time	What happened?	Where?	Who else was present?	What could be happening internally (*inside* client) to precipitate behavior?	What could be happening externally (*outside* client) to precipitate behavior?	What interventions help (could help) client?
							Camouflage tube by use of fitted underwear. Eliminate bulky dressing as soon as possible. Involve in diversional activity (likes books and magazines with pictures of flowers).

Strumpf, N. E., & Evans, L. K. (1994–1998). *Maintaining restraint reduction in nursing homes* (1 RO1 AGO 8324). Bethesda, MD: National Institute on Aging.

Appendix J

Behavior Log 3: Attempting to Pull Out Endotracheal Tube

Specific Behavior: Attempting to pull out endotracheal tube

Client's Name: M. Scott Room # 4208

Date	Exact time	What happened?	Where?	Who else was present?	What could be happening internally (*inside* client) to precipitate behavior?	What could be happening externally (*outside* client) to precipitate behavior?	What interventions help (could help) client?
5/24/98	4:00 AM	Adhesive tapes removed and pulling at endotracheal tube.	Hospital room.	RN, M. Miller.	Fearful of tube and ventilator. Discomfort. Anxiety when coughing/being suctioned.	Pressure on nares/oropharynx from ET tube. Trauma to nasal tissue. Dry oral cavity. NPO.	Explain reason for treatment. Explain equipment (ETT, AmbuBag, ventilator). Explain procedures (suctioning, chest percussion, etc.).

(continued)

Appendix J *(continued)*

Date	Exact time	What happened?	Where?	Who else was present?	What could be happening internally (*inside* client) to precipitate behavior?	What could be happening externally (*outside* client) to precipitate behavior?	What interventions help (could help) client?
						Adhesive tape securing ETT is uncomfortable. Ventilator alarms are disturbing/frightening. Environmental noise, lights, activity.	Provide nasal and oral care q shift & prn. Provide guided exploration. Use tube holder instead of adhesive tape to secure ETT. Provide analgesia sedation and avoid physical restraints. Involve in diversional activity (to extent possible.) Plan for family to be at bedside. Provide soothing, quiet music. Decrease environmental noise and lights. Use hand mitts or ski gloves if above efforts fail. Provide supervised trials without mitts or gloves as soon as feasible.

Strumpf, N. E., & Evans, L. K. (1994–1998). *Maintaining restraint reduction in nursing homes* (1 RO1 AGO 8324). Bethesda, MD: National Institute on Aging.

Appendix K

Behavior Log 4: Attempting to Loosen Tracheostomy Ties and Remove Dressing

Specific Behavior: Attempting to untie trach ties and remove dressing

Client's Name: M. Scott Room # 210

Date	Exact time	What happened?	Where?	Who else was present?	What could be happening internally (*inside* client) to precipitate behavior?	What could be happening externally (*outside* client) to precipitate behavior?	What interventions help (could help) client?
6/15/98	10:00 AM	Trach ties undone; dressing dislodged.	Resident's room.	CNA, J. Jenson in hall.	Discomfort and pain from ties that may be too tight. Anxiety when coughing.	Pressure on neck and carotids from ties. Excoriation/ irritation of skin around trach site.	Maintain secure but comfortable trach ties. Place protective pads under ties to prevent irritation of skin.

(continued)

Appendix K *(continued)*

Date	Exact time	What happened?	Where?	Who else was present?	What could be happening internally (*inside* client) to precipitate behavior?	What could be happening externally (*outside* client) to precipitate behavior?	What interventions help (could help) client?
					Discomfort due to soreness around trach stoma.	Mucus draining onto excoriated skin causing burning and discomfort. Corrugated tubing from T-piece may be too short, pulling at trach tube. Trach dressing may be soiled and malodorous or offensive.	Change trach dressings frequently. Check with resident to ensure comfort and flexibility of T-piece extension tubing. Provide suctioning frequently to keep airway clear. Involve in diversional activity (tapes, books, magazines, etc.). Promote visiting from family. Provide soothing, quiet music. Decrease environmental noise. Provide guided exploration. Use hand mitts or ski gloves if above efforts fail. Provide supervised trials without mitts/gloves ASAP.

Strumpf, N. E., & Evans, L. K. (1994–1998). *Maintaining restraint reduction in nursing homes* (1 RO1 AGO 8324). Bethesda, MD: National Institute on Aging.

7

Maintaining a Process of Change

Joan Stockman Wagner and Neville E. Strumpf

The Purpose of this Chapter is to:

Explore the process of change as it relates to implementation and institutionalization of individualized, restraint-free care.

I. Introduction

A. Restraint-free care is a goal for acute and long-term care institutions. Recognizing the need for change; unfreezing or breaking down myths, assumptions, and old habits and practices; and moving ahead to implement restraint-free care is only the beginning. Continuous effort is needed to support staff who have gained new knowledge and skills, if such individualized care is to be maintained.

B. Restraint-free care means improved quality of life for the client. Quality of life is defined by the individual but frequently includes:

1. Ability to maintain control through personal decisions and choices, especially as they concern everyday life.
2. Maintaining or establishing meaningful relationships.

3. Living in a comfortable and appropriate environment providing sufficient privacy.
4. Preservation of the greatest physical and psychosocial function possible.

These quality of life attributes cannot be realized when the resident/client is physically restrained.

C. Maintaining the change to restraint-free care involves:

1. Adopting an institution-wide philosophy of individualized care.
2. Knowing the negative consequences and effects of physical restraint.
3. Individualizing responses based on a systematic analysis of behavior.
4. Continuing education and modeling for all staff, with reinforcement of accomplishments:

   a. A philosophy of care, along with policies and procedures, clearly in place to guide staff toward restraint-free care.
   b. New attitudes, skills, knowledge, and practice patterns.
   c. Successful testimonials as solutions aimed at restraint-free care are implemented.

II. Review of Key Concepts

A. Philosophy of Individualized Care (Happ, Williams, Strumpf, & Burger, 1996).

1. Based on descriptions in the literature, individualized care is defined as an interdisciplinary approach to care which acknowledges each person as separate and unique. Individualized care is practiced through consistent caring relationships. Knowledge about the person is used to create a care environment and ways of living which are congruent with and maintain continuity in the person's past patterns of life and individual preferences. Individualized care seeks to bring comfort and joy to the older adult by building on strengths and pleasurable experiences. The goals of individualized care for the older adult are to:

   a. maintain identity and human relationships;
   b. promote autonomy and independent decision making; and
   c. promote participation in and direction of care.

2. Individualized care is dependent upon:

   a. *Getting to know the person* as an individual, family and community member. Getting to know the person involves not only recognizing immediate life situations but also obtaining the life history, an important step in understanding individual responses and behaviors, and empathizing with feelings.

b. The right to make *choices*. The right to make decisions affecting all aspects of life is important to individualized care. As adults, choices are made daily about food, clothing, and activities. We make choices related to our environment, our friends and our life work. Important to the concept of individualized care is respect for rights of older adults to accept risk as a part of normal living. The attainment and maintenance of optimal physical, psychosocial, and emotional functioning is contingent on reasonable risk taking.

c. Establishing *relationships*. Care providers become increasingly important in the life of frail older adults, especially in long-term care. Staff not only provide necessary physical and psychological care, but also become critical members of the older adult's social and emotional life. Appropriateness of and continuity in staff assignment to the older adult is essential to build and maintain positive and meaningful relationships.

d. *Resident participation and direction* of care. The older adult who is known as a unique individual, lives life in relationships with others, and has an active role in making personal choices, has the means of participating in and directing his/her own care. The older adult is a vital part of the decision-making team. Team members share information and concerns and discuss a plan of action. Through the decision making involved in directing care, older adults gain a measure of control that signifies dignity and responsibility.

B. Consequences and Effects of Physical Restraint

1. Numerous negative outcomes from use of physical restraint exist. Care providers who advocate physical restraint as a means to *protect the older adult from harm* should consider the potential untoward effects of restraint use related to physical, psychosocial, behavioral, and safety outcomes.
2. The application of physical restraints may actually risk *harm to* the older adult. The consequences can be devastating and may be irreversible.

C. Responses to Specific Behaviors

1. Systematic assessment.

a. Commitment to individualized care involves the completion of a comprehensive systematic assessment of the older adult. Performing this assessment assists the caregiver in getting to know the person in his/her world. The steps of such an assessment are outlined in chapter 3.

b. A systematic assessment assists in understanding the context or circumstances of the behavior(s), and allows care providers to respond to unmet needs and changes in health status

2. Interventions are most effective when they are individualized and in response to specific needs.

Identifying appropriate interventions to address health state change or to meet client needs requires creative problem solving. Interventions include:

a. Physiologic approaches.
b. Psychosocial approaches.
c. Activity and exercise programs.
d. Environmental modification.

Examples of interventions are found in Appendix A.

III. Supporting the Momentum

A. Continuing Education and Modeling for Staff

1. It is important to maintain the momentum once a restraint-free care program is operational. Staff have acquired new knowledge, skills and behaviors which need to become permanent. Continuous education and support are needed to maintain restraint-free care.

Staff need the opportunity to ask questions and collaborate with those individuals who are most knowledgeable about a restraint-free environment. These individuals serve as models and consultants by demonstrating and sharing skills in systematic assessment and responses to behaviors. Creative problem solving is key to the ongoing success of restraint-free care.

2. All new staff must be oriented to any program of restraint-free care. Education should, at a minimum, include:

a. Facility philosophy regarding restraint-free care.
b. Specific policies and procedures related to physical restraint .
c. Misconceptions about use of restraints.
d. Standards of care related to physical restraints.

e. Consequences and effects of restraint use.
f. Assessment guidelines for making sense of behavior.
g. Overview of responses to and interventions for specific behaviors.

New staff need support from other team members as they put new knowledge into clinical practice. Answering questions and assisting with problem solving are essential parts of the educational process.

3. Ongoing resident/client and family education is also important in supporting the momentum toward restraint-free care. Staff must take an active role in providing information and reassurance to both newly admitted clients and long-term residents and their families. Some risk taking is inherent in restraint-free care. Reassuring clients and families that staff will make every effort to reasonably provide for safety is essential. Clients should be educated about the consequences and effects of restraint use. The resident and family play a central role in individualizing care and should be encouraged to participate actively in problem solving. Informed clients and families clearly facilitate goals toward restraint-free care.

B. Testimonials of Success

Sharing "stories" of clients who have remained restraint free or who have had restraints eliminated is one way to help staff *celebrate their successes*. Success breeds enthusiasm and a desire to continue with efforts to achieve positive outcomes. Case presentations for unit staff are another way to support the momentum toward restraint-free care.

1. Clinical Example #1: Mr. J.

Mr. J. was admitted to the nursing facility post-CVA, aphasic, occasionally incontinent of urine, and with symptoms of multi-infarct dementia. He arrived with a PEG tube and limited lower extremity mobility. Mr. J. frequently pulled at his PEG tube, and when frustrated, would strike out at staff with a flailing arm motion.

A systematic assessment revealed that the site surrounding Mr. J.'s PEG tube was clean, dry and intact. Mr. J. did, however, pull back and appear fearful whenever the tube was handled. Staff also reported that Mr. J. seemed sensitive to loud noises and that his level of confusion and aggressiveness would increase with multiple stimuli in the environment. Mr. J. had been a high school teacher prior to his retirement and his family reported a lifetime interest in reading books about history.

Utilizing their observations and the above assessment data, the interdisciplinary team devised an individualized care plan which addressed Mr. J.'s needs. Staff believed that if Mr. J.'s comfort level could be increased and his anxiety decreased, he would be less likely to strike out at staff. To accomplish this:

a. A communication board was provided to assist Mr. J. in expressing his feelings and needs.
b. Staff greeted Mr. J. consistently by name and introduced themselves each time they approached him. Mr. J. responded very positively to this approach and his "striking out" behavior decreased significantly.
c. Staff assignments were consistent so that meaningful relationships could be developed, and care preferences could be established. Mr. J. was able to regain some control in his life.
d. A reclining chair was provided. Mr. J. appeared more comfortable and much happier with this seating arrangement. His recliner was often positioned near a window allowing a view of the world beyond his room.
e. A lateral support cushion was also used with his recliner, to help maintain an upright posture, further contributing to his comfort.
f. Staff were especially attentive to Mr. J.'s physical needs. His episodes of incontinence seemed especially stressful to him. Mr. J. was placed on a schedule for use of the toilet based on specific documented times for incontinence. This intervention not only contributed to an improvement in Mr. J.'s comfort level, but also appeared to decrease the frequency of "striking out."
g. Soft background music was provided and had noticeable calming effects.

Staff were also concerned that Mr. J. would injure himself by pulling at his PEG tube. To address these concerns, the team focused attention on providing distraction and meaningful activities for Mr. J. Interventions included:

a. Camouflage of the tube. This was accomplished by placing a thick dressing over the PEG tube and by tucking in shirt and sweater into pants, then fastening his belt.
b. Activities. Soft background music was also helpful in distracting attention from the PEG tube.

Mr. J. enjoyed 1:1 interaction with the activity therapist. He especially enjoyed having someone read to him or looking at picture books about history.

c. Trial oral feedings. After conferring with the physician and speech therapist, periodic trials of oral feeding were initiated. Attempts to eliminate the PEG tube were eventually successful.

Mr. J. did well with this individualized plan of care, which was developed collaboratively by Mr. J., his family, and the interdisciplinary team. Physical restraints were not used and the team felt very positive about the quality of care provided and the quality of life achieved for Mr. J.

2. Clinical Example #2: Mrs. S.

Mrs. S. was an 86-year-old resident admitted to a nursing facility for skilled care rehabilitation following repair of a left hip fracture. She was permitted only partial weight bearing. Mrs. S. sustained her fracture at home from a fall enroute to the bathroom. Mrs. S. had a history of recurrent heart failure and osteoarthritis. She had cataracts removed bilaterally and wore corrective eyeglasses. Mrs. S. was considered at risk for falls.

Mrs. S. had two near fall events on the evening shift at the skilled rehabilitation facility. Using a systematic approach, staff were able to better understand the nature of Mrs. S.'s near fall "events" and establish an individualized plan of care. Interviews with Mrs. S. revealed:

a. Both "events" happened between 4:00 and 6:00 p.m.
b. Both "events" happened when she was enroute to the bathroom
c. Mrs. S. was wearing her eyeglasses at the time of the first event.
d. At that time, she was attempting to get up from the green chair in her room, using her walker as support. She reported, "I just couldn't get up. When I finally did manage to stand, I lost my balance for a few seconds but managed to steady myself."
e. At the time of the second event, Mrs. S. had been resting in her bed before experiencing an "urgent" need to void. She reported, "I managed to get out of bed with some difficulty. I was halfway to the bathroom when my feet just slipped out from under me. I would have surely fallen if that dresser had not been there for me to grab onto." The nursing assistant had placed Mrs. S.'s glasses in her bedside drawer.

To understand the reasons for Mrs. S.'s near fall events further, the team listed the following additional internal and external factors:

a. Mrs. S. was receiving 40 mg. of Lasix b.i.d. for her heart failure. The last dose was scheduled for 2:00 p.m.

b. The nursing assistant reported that Mrs. S. was not wearing slippers or shoes at the time of the second event.
c. Mrs. S. has little depth perception, and loses her balance easily when not wearing her glasses.
d. The green chair in Mrs. S.'s room was low to the floor. Mrs. S. measured 5′8″ in height.
e. While Mrs. S. had been progressing with her physical therapy, she still needed a contact guard when using her walker. Mrs. S. did not always call for assistance.
f. Mrs. S. had been a homemaker and mother of six children. She had always been a very active woman, participating in church, school, and community projects. She attended a local senior center almost daily until about a year ago, when episodes of heart failure became more frequent. Mrs. S. realized that another fall could result in serious consequences for her. She was vehement, however, about her willingness to take some risk in order to maintain her highly valued independence.

Utilizing data from this assessment, a care plan was devised incorporating the following individualized approaches:

a. Mrs. S. was instructed to use her call bell for assistance before attempting ambulation. Her call bell was secured to her bed/chair for easy accessibility. Ability to follow instructions to call for assistance would be monitored and, if necessary, a bed/chair alarm system would be considered.
b. "Fall risk" code stickers were secured to her care plan and next to her room number on the call light box to alert staff to respond promptly.
c. A night light was used from early evening throughout the night to provide better visibility of the bedroom and bathroom environments.
d. Slippers with slip resistant soles were secured and kept at Mrs. S.'s bedside. Mrs. S. was educated about the importance of wearing slippers (or shoes) whenever ambulating.
e. Non-slip strips were applied to the floor next to her bed and in front of the toilet in the bathroom.
f. Staff were instructed to place Mrs. S.'s eyeglasses in their case and on top of her bedside stand whenever she took a nap and at bedtime. This action assisted Mrs. S. in finding her glasses promptly when needed.
g. Mrs. S.'s green room chair was replaced with a more appropriate chair which made it easier for her to rise safely and maintain her balance.
h. Mrs. S.'s lasix was rescheduled so that she received the required dosage in the morning. This helped to reduce her frequent trips to

the bathroom, often extending into the evening hours. She still experienced urgency until early afternoon, however, and was monitored closely.

i. A schedule was established for use of the toilet based on documented intervals of voiding as recorded on a voiding diary/log.

j. An inservice education session was conducted by the physical/occupational therapists to assist staff in providing the support necessary for safe transfers. Mrs. S.'s therapy sessions were continued and she progressively improved.

k. Mrs. S. enjoyed group activities. She especially enjoyed playing chair balloon volleyball and afternoon group classes where she could exercise her arms and upper torso to music. While she tired easily, these activities helped maintain Mrs. S.'s upper extremity strength and ultimately made use of her walker an easier task.

The use of physical restraints would have been devastating to this dignified and active woman. Furthermore, it is likely that use of physical restraints would have hindered Mrs. S.'s full rehabilitation and could even have contributed to permanent institutionalization or death. Mrs. S. returned to her home after 15 days of rehabilitation. Home care and therapy were prescribed post-discharge.

IV. Modifying Policy and Procedure Related to Restraint Use

Philosophically, a commitment to individualized restraint-free care should negate the need for polices and procedures related to physical restraint use. Realistically, however, even hospitals and nursing facilities supporting restraint-free care may have *extreme* occasions when a physical restraint will be applied on a short-term basis. In addition, at this moment in time, regulations governing hospitals and nursing homes require policies and procedures for restraint use.

A major task of an interdisciplinary restraint reduction committee/task force committed to restraint-free care is development or modification of policies and procedures related to physical restraints. These policies should be reviewed periodically, with modification as necessary to reflect current standards of practice. Policies and procedures should place emphasis on the goal of individualized restraint-free care. Highlighted below are a broad set of topics that should be addressed in facility policies and procedures related to physical restraint. It should be noted that the time required by staff to adhere to these policies is often more labor intensive, and certainly less satisfying for staff and the older adult than caring for patients/residents without restraints.

A. Philosophy of Care

1. To begin, review and, as necessary, modify the existing philosophy related to use of physical restraints. What are the facility and staff's beliefs about restraint? Is the goal to become restraint free or to limit the number/duration of restraints? Limiting restraints and changing to use of least restrictive devices may be a first goal, followed by total elimination. The long-term goal of restraint-free care is to improve or maintain function and improve quality of life and care for older adults. The use of physical restraints is incompatible with the goals of maximal function and quality of life.
2. Once the philosophy of care is in place, current policies can be revised and procedures outlined that are compatible with the new goals.

B. Policies and Procedures

1. Points to Address:

a. Definition of Restraint

- Definitions of restraint vary from facility to facility, and individual to individual. Definitions are also determined by federal and state regulations and accreditation guidelines.
- Be clear about what constitutes restraint. Some facilities use terms such as "safety device," "assistive device," or "medical immobilization." Use of these terms is confusing and may even promote the use of physical restraint.
- "Physical restraints" may be defined as:

> *. . . any manual method, physical or mechanical device, material, or equipment attached or adjacent to the resident's body that the individual cannot remove easily which restricts freedom of movement or normal access to one's body. Physical restraints include, but are not limited to, leg restraints, arm restraints, hand mitts, soft ties or vests, lap cushions and lap trays the resident cannot remove. Likewise, wheelchair safety bars, chairs/gerichairs, and bed rails that prevent the resident from voluntarily rising are considered physical restraints.* (HCFA, 1992 Interpretive Guidelines 483.13(a)

- It is recommended that staff consult regularly for any changes in relevant restraint definitions and guidelines, e.g., from the Healthcare Financing Administration, Joint Commission on Accreditation of Health Care Organizations, etc.

b. Informed Consent for Clients and Families

- Philosophy and policies regarding restraint use should be shared with potential residents, patients, and family prior to admission.
- If policy permits restraint use in emergency or specified situations, client and family need to be informed about options.
- The policy should indicate the mechanisms by which clients and families are told of potentially harmful consequences of restraint use. Some facilities have a consent form to be signed by the client if a physical restraint is to be used, noting type of restraint to be applied; the reason for the restraint; and possible consequences of restraint application.
- A policy should consider situations where decisional incapacity exists, defining the role of family members or the legal representative.

c. Preventive Strategies

1. Assessment - See Chapter 3.
2. Interventions - Examples are found in Appendix A.

d. Circumstances for Use and Emergency Procedures
e. Initiation and Application by Whom
f. Procedures During Restraint Use and for Release or Removal
g. Plans for Re-evaluation
h. Nursing Responsibilities Regarding Interventions

Policies and procedures should describe nursing responsibilities relating to:

1. Comprehensive assessment of the individual
2. Collaborative decision making regarding non-restrictive approaches which might be appropriate, and documentation of the decision not to restrain or to restrain
3. Involvement of the client/legal representative
4. Maintenance of human dignity

i. Documentation by Team Members

Documentation should be addressed in the policies and procedures and include:

1. A detailed physician order.
2. Assessment.
3. Evidence of interdisciplinary collaboration.

(a) written summary from the interdisciplinary team meeting
(b) nursing or rehabilitation consultation
(c) physical or occupational therapy evaluation
(d) mental health consultation

4. Informed consent
5. Interventions

2. *The thrust of all policies and procedures should clearly uphold a standard of restraint-free care.*

C. Resources (Refer to Appendix B)

Further information about resources for restraint-free care are listed. These are *not* substitutes for assessment, individualized care planning, ongoing evaluation, and support. They are but a tiny part in a much larger cultural change.

Bibliography

An ongoing problem: Restraints and time-limited orders. (1996). *Briefings of JCAHO*, No. 1996, p. 6–12.

Braun, J. (1993). Preparing for implementation. *In Toward a Restraint Free Environment.* Baltimore, MD: *Health Professions Press,* 11–29.

Brower, T. (1991). The alternatives to restraints. *Journal of Gerontological Nursing, 17*(2), 18–22.

Cutchins, C. (1991). Blueprint for restraint-free care. *American Journal of Nursing, 91*(7), 36–42.

Elon, R., & Pawlson, L. G. (1992). The impact of OBRA on medial practice within nursing facilities. *Journal of the American Geriatrics Society, 40*(9), 958–963.

Feeney-Mahoney, D. (1995). Analyses of restraint free nursing homes. *Image: Journal of Nursing Scholarship, 27*(2), 155–160.

Happ, M. B., Williams, C., Strumpf, N., & Burger, S. (1996). Individualized care for frail elders: Theory and practice. *Journal of Gerontological Nursing, 22*(3), 7–13.

Harris, E., & Fehr, S. (1992). A journey to restraint-free care. *Untie the Elderly, 4*(2), 1–6.

Healthcare Financing Administration. (1992). *The Long Term Care Survey.* Washington, DC: American Health Care Association.

Joint Commission on Accreditation of Healthcare Organizations. (1996). *Restraint and seclusion: Addressing the issues/complying with the standards.* Oakbrook Terrace, IL: JCAHO.

Joint Commission on Accreditation of Healthcare Organizations. (1996). *Restraint and seclusion: A new approach for hospitals.* Oakbrook-Terrace, IL: JCAHO.

Joint Commission on Accreditation of Healthcare Organizations (1997). *Comprehensive Accreditation Manual for Hospitals: The official handbook.* Oakbrook-Terrace, IL: JCAHO

Katims, I. (1995). The contrary ideals of individualism and nursing values of care. *Scholarly Inquiry for Nursing Practice, 9*(3), 231–240.

Kayser-Jones, J. (1992). Culture, environment, and restraints: A conceptual model for research and practice. *Journal of Gerontological Nursing, 18*(11), 13–20.

Koroknay, V. (1993). Implementing a restraint removal program. In *Toward a restraint free environment.* Baltimore, MD: Health Professions Press, 53–60.

Koroknay, V., Braun, J., & Lipson, S. (1993). Educating staff, residents, and families about restraint reduction. In *Toward a restraint free environment.* Baltimore, MD: Health Professions Press, 31–45.

Morrison, J., Crinklaw, D., King, D., Thibeault, S., & Wells, D. (1987). Formulating a restraint use policy. *Journal of Nursing Administration, 17*(3), 39–42.

Patterson, J., Strumpf, N., & Evans, L. (1995). Nursing consultation to reduce restraints in a nursing home. *Clinical Nurse Specialist, 9*(4), 213–235.

Schnelle, J. F., Ouslander, J. G., & Cruise, P. A. (1997). Policy without technology: A barrier to improving nursing home care. *The Gerontologist, 37*(4), 527–532.

Siegler, E., Capezuti, E., Maislin, G., Baumgarten, M., Evans, L., & Strumpf, N. (1997). Effects of a restraint reduction intervention and OBRA '87 regulations on psychoactive drug use in nursing homes. *Journal of the American Geriatrics Society, 45*, 791–796.

Special Report: Restraint and Seclusion Standards. *Joint Commission Perspectives*, Jan/Feb 1996, p. 21–26.

Strumpf, N. E. (1997). Achieving restraint-free care in hospital settings. *Untie the Elderly, 9*(3), 1–3.

Appendix A

Matrix of Behaviors and Interventions

Types of Interventions	Fall Risk	Treatment Interference	Other Behaviors
Physiologic	• Identification of reasons for falling and comprehensive assessment • Medication review/elimination of troublesome drugs • Evaluation and prescription for PT/OT, etc. • Rest • Elimination schedule	• Comfort • Pain relief • Assistance with elimination • Evaluation of need for change in treatment (e.g., remove IV/NG tubes, catheters, wean from ventilator)	• Comfort • Pain relief • Correction of underlying problem, e.g. dehydration • Positioning • Attention/assistance with elimination • Sensory aids • Massage/aroma therapy

(continued)

Appendix A *(continued)*

Types of Interventions	Fall Risk	Treatment Interference	Other Behaviors
Psychosocial	• Supervision • Authorization of "no restraint" from resident/family • Fall/risk program • Anticipation of needs	• Companionship and supervision • Authorization of "no re-straint" from resident/family • Encouragement of appropriate advance directive • Reassurance • Maintenance of communication with family/ resident • Ethics consult as indicated	• Companionship • Therapeutic touch • Active listening • Calm approach • Provision of sense of safety and security/validation of concerns • "Timeout" PRN • Care-giver consistency • Supervision • Promotion of trust and sense of purpose/mastery • Attention to resident's agenda • Reality orientation (if appropriate) • Remotivation • Attention to feelings and concerns • Facilitation of resident control over activities of daily living • Pastoral/spiritual counseling • Family visits and information sharing • Communications that are calm, sensitive to cues, and use simple statements/instructions
Activities	• Daily physical therapy/ambula-tion/weight bearing • Gait training • Fall-prevention program • Transfer assistance • Restorative program • Meaningful activity	• Distraction • Television, ra-dio, music • Something to hold	• Distraction • Planned recreation (consistent with interest/abilities) • Exercise • PT/OT/ADL training • Social activity • Outlets for anxious behavior, especially structured activity • Nighttime activities PRN • Redirection toward unit • Pet therapy • Structured routines • Spiritual activities and outlets

(continued)

Appendix A *(continued)*

Types of Interventions	Fall Risk	Treatment Interference	Other Behaviors
Environmental	• Chairs that slant or fit body, wedge cushions, abductor pillow or other customized seating • Low beds, bed rails down or single side rails, pads, accessible call light, mattress on floor, bedside commode, table placed in front of chair • Mobility aids and supportive shoes • Safety awareness training, fall-safe environment, alarm signal system, assistive devices, elevated toilet seat • Varied sitting locations • Optimal lighting	• Placement near nursing station • Accessible call light • Camouflaged or padded treatment site • Protective sleeves, garments, etc.	• Decreased use of intercom • Decreased/increased light as appropriate • Quiet room or soothing background music/rocking chair • Personalized area/homelike environment/familiar objects • Camouflaged doors, exits, elevators • Floor tape (grids) or planters to signal end of hall • Special locks • Alarm systems • Contained areas that are safe and interesting • Special clothing • Varied seating and furnishings • Personal space • Structured environment • Room change as appropriate

Appendix B

Resources

The following list of resources, including general information and equipment, is compiled to assist those engaged in the implementation of restraint-free care. It is important to stress, however, that a philosophy of individualized care requires far more than the use of products to replace physical restraints. As has been emphasized throughout this clinical guide, restraint-free care comes about as a process of commitment to the assessment of individual needs and the application of interventions specifically tailored to meet those needs. Although the following list may provide helpful leads and directions, it is *not* exhaustive. In addition, it is not an endorsement of any of the products, equipment, or companies that have been included, and we do not have any product-testing information available.

General Information

Books and Workbooks

1. "Retrain, Don't Restrain," a guide to restraint reduction for clinical coordinators. Available with trainer's manual, workbooks and videotape. Developed by the Jewish Home and Hospital for the Aged. American Health Care Association, Publications Department B1, PO Box 96906, Washington, DC: 20090-6906 or AAHSA at 800-508-9442.
2. "Toward a Restraint-Free Environment" by J. Braun, and S. Lipson. Health Professions Press, PO Box 10624, Baltimore, MD: 21285-0624. 888-337-8808.
3. "Surveyors Study Guide to Chemical and Physical Restraint Avoidance in Long Term Care Facilities." Produced by the Health Care Financing Administration. Distributed by NTIS, U.S. Dept. Of Commerce, Springfield, VA: 22161. 703-487-4650. Product #: 19918VNB1.
4. "Life-Enhancing Activities for Mentally Impaired Elders" by Beverly Ann Beisgen. Springer Publishing, 536 Broadway, 11th floor, NY, NY: 10012. 212-431-4370.

5. "Doing Things" by J.M. Zgola. A book describing activities suitable for persons with low cognitive functioning. Johns Hopkins University Press, Hampdon Station, Baltimore, MD: 21211. 410-516-6956.
6. "Holding On To Home: Designing Environments for People with Dementia" by U. Cohen and G.D. Weisman. Johns Hopkins University Press, Hampdon Station, Baltimore, MD: 21211. 410-516-6956.
7. "Individualized Dementia Care: Creative, Compassionate Approaches." Joanne Rader and Elizabeth Tornquist. Appendix F highlights resources available to caregivers. Springer Publishing, 536 Broadway, 11th floor, NY, NY: 10012. 212-431-4370.

Media

1. "Proper Use of Restraints: A Balancing Act," video and workbook. "Problems, benefits and alternatives to restraints are discussed from the point of view of administrators, nurses, medical directors, occupational therapists and activity professionals." American College of Health Care Administrators (ACHCA), 325 S. Patrick St., Alexandria, VA: 22314. 703-549-5822.
2. "Choice Among Risks: Physical Restraints Rejected"—a video by Montefiore Medical Center, Bronx, N.Y. Distributed by Health Professions Press, PO Box 10624, Baltimore, MD: 21285-0624. 888-337-8808.
3. "How to be a Nurse Assistant." Pro-Care Interactive Video Disk Training. Interactive Health Network, 17 Executive Parkway, Suite 250, Atlanta, GA: 30327.
4. "Physical Restraints: Innovative Solutions to Restraint Reduction." Video describing "the physician's role, responsibilities, and options under the regulations resulting from OBRA '87." ADMA, 10480 Little Patuxent Pkwy., S#760, Columbia, MD: 21044. 410-740-9743. FAX: 410-740-4572.
5. "Restraint-Free Care and the Environment: Scenes from a Swedish Nursing Home." Gerontological Nursing Consultation Service, University of Pennsylvania School of Nursing, Ralston House, 3615 Chestnut St., Philadelphia, PA: 215-898-4998. Contact person: Becky Phillips.
6. "Designing the Physical Environment for Persons with Dementia." Terra Nova Films, 9848 S. Winchester, Chicago, IL: 60643. 773-881-8491.

Newsletters

1. Restraint-free newsletter, "Untie the Elderly," published quarterly (address requests to Untie the Elderly or to Mary Scharf). Also available are many related resources including videos such as "Everyone Wins! Quality Care Without Restraints," a monograph entitled "Staff Attitudes on the Use and Elimination of Physical Restraints," and "Untie the Elderly Resource Manual." Kendal Corporation, PO Box 100, Kennett Square, PA: 19348. 610-388-7001. Or e mail (www.ute.kendal.org).

2. National Citizens' Coalition for Nursing Home Reform publishes an excellent newsletter, "Quality Care Advocate," as well as "Avoiding Physical Restraint Use: New Standards in Care". Other resource materials on physical and chemical restraints are available at modest cost. NCCNHR, 1424 16th St., NW, Suite 202, Washington, DC: 20036; 202-332-2275.

Other

1. "Fall Sensing Evaluation Criteria." Prepared by Josef Osterweil, PhD. (Ph: 703-818-3951 or FAX: 301-460-4998)

Products

Alarms

1. "Wanderguard" wrist/ankle band signaling device. Door or overhead monitors give visual and auditory alarm on site when patient crosses area. "Tabs Mobility Monitor" for use with chair, bed or wheelchair. Alarms when wearer moves beyond safety zone. Senior Technologies, 1550 N. 20th Circle, Lincoln, NE: 68503. 800-824-2996.
2. "Care Trak" for monitoring and locating wanderers. Mobile locator with wrist alarm for patient as well as perimeter and building alarm systems. 1031 Autumn Ridge Rd., Carbondale, IL: 62901. 800-842-4537 or 618-549-2356. FAX: 618-457-3340.
3. "Ambualarm" and "chair sensor" for detecting movement to a vertical position. 30 day free trial period. Alert Care, 591 Redwood Highway, Suite 2125, Mill Valley, CA: 94941. 800-826-7444.
4. "Bed Check" and "Chair Check" monitoring systems. Bed Check Corp., Box 170, Tulsa, OK: 74101-0170. 800-523-7956.
5. "Code Alert." Pressure change alarm for bed or chair. RF Technologies, 3125 N. 126th St., Brookfield, WI: 53005. 800-669-9946.
6. "Patriot Alarm." Alerts caregiver to position change. Safety Technology, International, Inc., 2306 Airport Rd., Waterford, MI: 48327. 800-888-4784.

Beds and Bed Products

1. Low beds—spring height < 13 inches. Specialty "Lo Max" model is 4.5 inches from the floor without casters. Some models have dual controls. Half-side rails also available. "Designed Perimeter Mattress" has foam ridge down both sides. NM Industries, 2935 N. Parkway, Atlanta, GA: 30360. 800-554-9224.
2. Low beds including "Alzheimer's Bed." Basic American Medical—Omni Division, 2935 Bankers Industrial Dr., Atlanta, GA: 30360.

3. Gel-filled "Flotation Cushions" by Spinal Technologies, 1940 Rutgers Blv., Lakewood, NJ: 09701. 800-257-5145.
4. Low beds and beds without side rails; overbed tables with rims. J. Nesbit Evans and Company, Ltd., Wooden Road West, Wednesbury, West Midlands, WS10 7BL, United Kingdom. 021-556-1511. Telex: 339123 (NESBIT G).
5. NOA Riser Bed (adjusts from standard bed height of 23 in. down to 7 in. above the floor). NOA Medical Industries, Inc., 205 N. Two St. Marthasville, MO: 66357. 888-662-6699.
6. Low beds. Gem Industries, PO Box 610, Toccoa, GA: 30577. Ph: 706-886-8431. FAX: 706-886-5119.

Seating

1. Recliner, bath and shower seats, commodes, transfer benches, etc. Lumex, 100 Spence St., Bayshore, NY: 11706-2290. 800-645-5272. FAX: 800-545-8639.
2. "Safety Seat." An insert to prevent user from sliding forward in chair or wheelchair. Davi Corporation, Department GN, Box 1016, Belgrade, MT: 59714. 406-282-7433.
3. Contoured, specialized seating—numerous products and models. Also available, portable devices for sensory stimulation. Kirton Products, 23 Rockwood Way, Hollands Road Industrial Estate, Haverhill, Suffolk CB9 8PB, England. (0440) 705352. Fax: (0440) 706199.
4. Lounge chair with safety sides, "Johnson D-Placement Cushion," "Cheese Leaner," foot lifts. Ask for Restraint Alternative Catalogue. Clock Medical Supply, 901 Industrial Rd., Winfield, KA: 67156. 316-221-0550.
5. Seat cushions, wheelchair inserts, narrow bolsters, back supports, wedges, footrest extender and elevation kits, lateral support cushions, etc. Alimed Inc., 297 High St., Dedham, MA: 02026-2839. 800-225-2610. http://www.alimed.com
6. Transfer discs, 12 inch and 15 inch."Sit Straight" and wedge cushions, soft splints. Sammons-Preston, Box 5071, Bolingbrook, IL: 60440-5071. 800-323-5547.
7. Anti-tipping devices for wheel chairs and walkers. Invacare Corp., 899 Cleveland St., PO Box 4028, Elyria, OH: 44036-2125; 800-INVACARE.
8. Olympic Medical Vac-Pac Positioning System. Pads containing plastic beads moulded into position by vacuum. Pads can be remoulded for each use. 5900 1st Av. South, Seattle, WA: 98108. 800-426-0353.
9. "Fallout Chair" constructed of high density foam. "Incontinent-proof" with lumbar, head, and neck support. QFoam International, Canada, Custom Foam Systems, Ltd., 360 Trillium Dr., Kitschener, Ontario, Canada, N2E2K6. 519-748-1700. FAX: 519-748-0936. Distributor: Brad Miller: 800-569-9992.

10. Seating cushions. Skil-Care. 29 Wells Av., Yonkers, NY: 10701. 800-431-2972.
11. Specialized seating. Hill-Rom, 1069 State Route 46 E, Batesville, IN: 47006-9167. 812-934-7777.
12. Specialized, adjustable seating. Skandi-Form AB, S-288 34 Vinslov, Sweden. 044-855 50. U.S. distributor: Design Link, International, 25 Kingston St. Boston, MA: 02111. 617-451-9050.
13. Inflatable seat cushions. Roho, 100 N. Florida Av., Belleville, IL: 62221. 800-851-3449.
14. "Litenest." A seat with back, multidensity foam pad. Better Body Co., 8339 S. Hindrey Av., Los Angeles, CA: 90045. 800-432-2225.
15. Seats, cushions and backs. Jay Medical, Ltd., 7477A Dry Creek Parkway, Longmont, CO: 80503. 800-648-8282.
16. "Ultraform" wedge cushion prevents sliding and lessens pressure. American Health Systems, Inc., P.O. Box 26688, Greenville, SC: 29616-1688. 800-234-6655.
17. "Varilite" inflatable chair cushions conform to the individual to correct posture problems. Cascade Designs, Inc., 4000 1st Av., S., Seattle, WA: 98134. 800-527-1527.
18. Carolina Rocker, helps convert wheel chair to rocker. ARTEC, Inc., P.O. Box 25103, Greenville, SC: 29616. 803-288-2111.
19. "Life-Ride" chair facilitates transfers and converts to a walker. Arjo, Inc., 8130 Lehigh Av., Morton Grove, IL: 60053. 800-323-1245.
20. Customized seating, including the Flemming system, and positioning cushions. Global Industries, 17 West Stowe Rd., Marlton, NJ: 08053. 609-596-3390.
21. Positioning cushions for bed, chair, and wheelchair; "Orthotic Seating System" and self-release belts. J.T. Posey Co., 5635 Peck Rd., Arcadia, CA: 91006-0020. 818-443-3143.

Diversions

1. "Tub of Fun," containing recreational products for persons with dementia. Included are items for sensory stimulation, manipulation and communication. Among these are sewing cards, "The Tangle," and dolls. Cross Creek Recreational Products, Inc., P.O. Box 289, Millbrook, NY: 12545. 914-677-9513.
2. "Discovery Aprons"—individually-made aprons containing buckles, zippers, buttons, materials for tactile stimulation, etc. to occupy patients with dementia. Potentials Development, Inc., 40 Hazelwood Dr., Suite 100, Amherst, NY: 14228. 716-691-6601.
3. "Bedscapes." Around-bed curtains imprinted with nature scenes and accompanying recordings of natural sounds. Bedscapes International, 146 Spencer Rd., Woodstock, NY: 12498. 914-657-8300.

4. Sense-stimulation products for patients with dementia including bells, wooden beads, aroma therapy products, and plastic sculpture kit. Geriatric Resources, Inc. P.O Box 239, Radium Springs, NM: 88054-0239. 800-359-0390.

Specialized Equipment

1. Velcro-release holders for tracheostomy and endotracheal tubes and for oxygen cannulas and central lines to prevent their removal. Dale Medical Co., 7 Cross St., Plainsville, MA: 02762. 800-343-3980. FAX: 508-695-6587.
2. "Flexi-Trak" anchoring devices for IV tubes, G and J tubes, indwelling catheters, pacemaker wires, etc. Convatech, 100 Headquarters Park Dr. Skillman, NJ: 08558. 908-281-2200.
3. "Doorguard," visual barrier made of vinyl to limit wandering. Bussard & Son, Inc. 415 25th Av., SW, Albany, OR: 97321. 541-926-7747.
4. "Rover" walkers with hand brakes. Noble Motion, Inc., PO Box 5366, Pittsburgh, PA: 15206-0366. 800-234-9255.
5. Raised toilet seats, positioning cushions, tube holders. Total Care, 18954 Bonanza Way, Gaithersburg, MD: 20879-1512. 800-334-3802.
6. "Fall-EZ" mat. Reduces fall related injuries. District Medical Supplies, 132 Cathedral St., Elkton, MD: 21921. 410-398-0555.
7. "Dignified products for dignified people." Dignit Ease, Inc., 8149 Ridge Ave., Philadelphia, PA: 19128. Ph/FAX: 215-483-4009.

Thanks to Joan Dunbar and Joanne Rader of the Restraint Free Task Force of the Gerontological Society of America, and The Delaware County (PA) Office of Services for the Aging, for their contributions to the above list.

Index